Drug Treatment in Gynaec

Second edition

Rodney S. Ledward, BSc, DA, MB, ChB, LRCP, MRCS, MRSH, DM, FRCS, FRCOG, DHMSA, MRPharm Soc.
Consultant Obstetrician and Gynaecologist, South East Kent Health Authority, William Harvey Hospital, Ashford, Kent, UK TN2 4OL

and

Stephen Cruikshank, MD
Chairman and Programme Director, Nicholas J Thompson Professor, Wright State University, Department of Obstetrics and Gynaecology, Miami Valley Hospital, Dayton, Ohio, USA.

with a Foreword by

Gedis Grudzinskas, MD, FRCOG
Professor, Department of Obstetrics and Gynaecology, The Royal London Hospital (Whitechapel), 4th Floor, Holland Wing, London E1 1BB

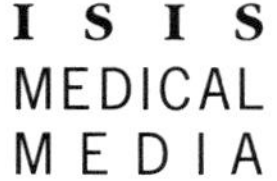
ISIS MEDICAL MEDIA

Oxford

Saxon Beck, 58 St Aldates
Oxford OX1 1ST, UK

First published 1984 by Butterworths & Co. (Publishers) Ltd
Second edition 1995 by Isis Medical Media Ltd

British Library Cataloguing in Publication Data
A catalogue record for this title is available from the British Library

ISBN 1 899066 04 7

Ledward R.S. (Rodney)
Drug Treatment in Gynaecology (second edition)/
Rodney Ledward and Stephen Cruikshank

Always refer to the manufacturer's Prescribing Information before prescribing drugs cited in this book.

Design and typesetting
Creative Associates, Oxford, UK

Printed by
Henry Ling Limited, Dorchester, UK

Distributors
Times Mirror International Publishers
Customer Service Centre, Unit 1, 3 Sheldon Way
Larkfield, Aylesford, Kent, ME20 6SF,
UK

Contents

Abbreviations

BNF	=	British National Formulary
BP	=	British Pharmacopoeia
BPC	=	British Pharmaceutical Codex
Eur. P	=	European Pharmacopoeia
USNF	=	United States National Formulary
USP	=	United States Pharmacopeia
CNS	=	Central Nervous System

Foreword (First edition)

In 1983 Mr Ledward, together with Professor Hawkins, published a handbook on drug therapy in obstetrics. This present book, written solely by Mr Ledward, is the companion volume on drug therapy in gynaecology. One of the major problems that confronts the young clinician is to remember the details and hazards of drug therapy in the various specialities that crowd the undergraduate curriculum. The emphasis tends to be laid on diagnosis rather than therapy, and yet gynaecological conditions which form a major part of general practice are often amenable to relatively simple therapeutic guidelines.

Having established the diagnosis, there is a need to identity and establish both the most appropriate therapy that is available and the relative risks and benefits that any particular treatment carries. This book seems to achieve those objectives in a concise and convenient manner. The subjects covered include those drugs used in the management of all common gynaecological disorders including pelvic infections, disorders of function such as premenstrual tension, dysmenorrhoea and dysfunctional uterine bleeding, and the management of organic disorders such as endometriosis and pelvic malignancies. The range of subjects is wide and the descriptions of management are, of necessity, brief. Nevertheless, the author has made a serious and, I believe, successful attempt to condense the essence of drug therapy in these disorders into a comprehensible and readily available format.

I recommend this book to all clinicians involved in the practice of gynaecological medicine as a concise and practical manual for drug therapy of gynaecological disorders.

E. M. Symonds, MD, FRCOG
Professor of Obstetrics and
Gynaecology, University of
Nottingham

Foreword (Second edition)

In the 10 years since the publication of the first edition of "Drug Treatment in Gynaecology", substantial advances and changes have occurred in the diagnosis and treatment of gynaecological disorders. These changes have occurred as a consequence of better understanding of human reproduction, the development of safer and more effective drugs and new strategies in the medical and surgical treatment of common disorders such as pelvic pain and menorrhagia.

The second edition has been revised to include new developments in drug therapy with particular relevance to the use in specific gynaecological disorders. The disorders in which the most substantial changes in practice have occurred include menorrhagia and dysfunctional uterine bleeding, endometriosis, uterine fibroids and infertility. The reader has brought up-to-date here the principles of usage of the new effective powerful drugs which have resulted in more effective treatment of these disorders without recourse of surgery.

Like my predecessor, I recommend this edition to all clinicians as a concise and practical book for drug therapy of gynaecological disorders.

Professor J G Grudzinskas
BSc, MB BS, MD, FRACOG, FRCOG

Preface (First edition)

This book is a gynaecological formulary based on its sister volume *Drug Treatment in Obstetrics* (Chapman and Hall, 1983). It provides specific prescribing information on the drugs most commonly used in gynaecological practice and will be a readily available source for resident gynaecological staff, family practitioners and gynaecological nursing staff. I hope it will also be of value to students reading for their final examinations and for their higher diplomas, and also for pharmacists.

In most sections, only drugs of known safety and proven efficacy are included. Practitioners are under pressure to prescribe the newest drugs, but these may not necessarily show any improvement on available drugs and potential side effects may not have presented. Practitioners should remain alert to the potential hazards of drugs and report such side effects to the Committee on Safety of Medicines. In many hospitals, prescribing guidance is provided by Drug and Therapeutics Committees. Expensive antibiotic prescribing is normally monitored by the consultant microbiologist, who may provide 'Guidelines in Antibiotic Prescribing' manuscripts.

The premenstrual syndrome illustrates *par excellence* that there is more to therapeutics than the use of drugs. A full explanation of any condition as is known is mandatory, together with reassurance, rest at home, diet, nursing care and physiotherapy and minimal use of drugs.

In certain sections of this book, reference is made to pregnancy simply because every woman (especially in the reproductive years) should be considered pregnant until proved otherwise, and potential teratogenic effects on an early and unsuspected pregnancy should be remembered.

Practitioners in obstetrics and gynaecology do not need to use a large armamentarium of preparations. They should aim to be thoroughly familiar with an adequate number of drugs rather than be unsure of many drugs, and this book has been written to allow the doctor to concentrate on those preparations in frequent use. References are included for further reading.

The completion of the book has been aided by the cooperation, encouragement and help of many friends, and my grateful thanks are extended to Malcolm Symonds, Professor of Obstetrics and Gynaecology at the University of Nottingham for writing the Foreword; Mr Trevor Lowenhoff, Principal

Pharmacist, Mayday Hospital, Croydon, for his help with the Drug Index and Glossary and general review of the manuscript; Dr Angela Dunham of the Department of Obstetrics and Gynaecology, South East Kent Health Authority for reading the proofs; Mrs Jean Gibson for typing the drafts; and to the staff of Butterworths for being such pleasant and patient colleagues.

Rodney S. Ledward

Preface (Second edition)

This book is an updated edition of *Drug Treatment in Gynaecology* first produced in 1984.

There have been many additions and changes since the first edition, not the least with gonadotrophin-releasing hormones and hormone-replacement therapy.

The format remains the same and it is hoped it will prove of help to residents, general practitioners and others actively engaged in prescribing.

Whilst small, no book is completed without the help and encouragement of many friends and I am extremely grateful to Professor Gedis Grudzinskas of The Royal London Hospital (Whitechapel) for writing the Foreword; to David Moloney, Principal Pharmacist of the South East Kent Health Authority for his help with reading the text and also to Mr Geoffrey Kumi, Staff Grade doctor, South East Kent Health Authority for similarly reviewing it; to Christine Andrews and Pamela Woodcock of South East Kent Health Authority who kindly typed the draft; and to Stephen Cruikshank who very kindly contributed to the book to ensure a North American input. I also record my thanks to Dr Stewart Coltart, Consultant Oncologist in the South East Kent Health Authority for editing the second appendix on oncological drugs.

The protocols for abortion and oncology differ so widely between the United Kingdom and the United States that both these topics have been placed in the appendices.

Finally, it has been a pleasure to acknowledge the support of John Harrison and Julian Grover of Isis Medical Media.

Rodney S. Ledward

Chapter 1

Vaginal Discharge

Introduction

The numerous types of vaginitis and causes of vaginal discharge include the following:

Physiological

1. Vulvovaginitis in childhood.
2. Leucorrhea — non-inflammatory discharge with negative microbiology.

Pathological

3. Infections:
   a. due to specific organisms, including *Candida*, *Chlamydia*, *Trichomonas* and *Neisseria* (gonorrhoea);
   b. Bacterial vaginosis
   c. chronic infections such as tuberculosis and syphilis.
4. Discharge from the cervix (erosions, polypi or carcinomas) and corpus uteri (polypi, carcinomas and endometritis).
5. Traumatic, including granulation tissue following hysterectomy.
6. Foreign bodies, including retained tampons and vaginal pessaries used to control prolapse.
7. Reactionary to douching or allergies to contraceptive rubber condoms or diaphragms.
8. Post-menopausal or atrophic vaginitis.

Sexual permissiveness is associated with an increase in trichomonal and gonorrhoeal infection; both infections should be excluded by laboratory tests and sexual partners treated concurrently if either infection is found. Fortunately, more specific venereal diseases such as syphilis are now relatively rare in the UK, but viral infections including herpes genitalis are appearing. If there is a clinical suspicion of possible venereal infection, patients should be questioned directly and all partners referred for further investigation at the local special venereal clinic.

There is an increasing incidence of candidiasis associated with the wider use of oral contraceptives, broad-spectrum antibiotics and the wearing of tights. It is also associated with diabetes mellitus and pregnancy.

With the advent of the imidazole derivatives, a major new class of antifungal drugs emerged, combining low toxicity and versatility of administration with a wide spectrum of antifungal action against dermatophytes, yeasts and dimorphic fungi. All azoles act on the P450 cytochrome enzyme and inhibit methylation of lanosterol, the predominant sterol of the fungal cell wall. This leads to deterioration of the membranes, uncontrolled cell-wall synthesis and a fungistatic or fungicidal effect.

Imidazoles also inhibit the transformation of *Candida* yeast to hyphal forms, which renders the organism more susceptible to phagocytosis by host leucocytes. The imidazoles include clotrimazole, miconazole, econazole, isoconazole and ketoconazole, and more recently itraconazole and fluconazole, and applications include pessaries, dusting powder, creams, medicated tampons and oral preparations.

Preparations used in the management of vaginal discharge and considered safe to be used during pregnancy include:

Acetic acid (to maintain a physiological vaginal pH of 4)
Lactic acid
Clotrimazole
Metronidazole
Miconazole nitrate
Nystatin
Penicillins
Povidone-iodine

Acceptable good clinical practice should ensure that no preparation is used without a proven clinical and bacteriological diagnosis — occasionally a vaginal discharge may be secondary to gynaecological malignancy such as carcinoma of the cervix.

Candida albicans (Thrush)

There is a growing incidence of this common infection with 75% of women affected at least once in their lifetime. It is associated with a thick curd-like white itchy discharge. Vulval soreness and vaginitis are common. It may be severe enough to cause sexual dysfunction and marital discord. Most women who suffer from thrush are healthy, but patients with diabetes mellitus or who are being treated with immunosuppressants or antibiotics or who may be taking oral contraceptive pills are particularly at risk. The diagnosis may be made on clinical grounds and confirmed by microscopic examination of a Gram-stained slide for yeast cells. Successful treatment is dependent on patient compliance and it is important to ensure that the full course of therapy is adhered to, even if the external signs (pruritus and discharge) have resolved. This is particularly important in pregnancy, where reports have indicated that, because the predisposing factors last until the end of pregnancy, eradication of the organism is consequently more difficult. The gut holds a reservoir of *Candida* as a commensal which may colonize the vagina as a pathogen if conditions prevail to encourage pathogenicity; systemic agents will treat reservoirs of *Candida* and reduce recurrence.

It is necessary to advise patients not to wear ordinary tights, to use underwear that can be boiled or to use disposable underwear. Daily bathing in warm water and the use of bland soaps should be recommended.

The ideal antimycotic suitable for all patients and all cases of vaginal candidiasis should have the following characteristics:

Short treatment course
Oral agent
Lack of local or systemic side effects and toxicity
Rapid action
Fungicidal
Minimal effect on normal bacterial flora of vagina
Safe in pregnancy
Reduced recurrence rate

Unfortunately potential litigation restricts the use of oral agents during pregnancies and topical agents should be initially prescribed.

Systemic preparations

Fluconazole

This is a bis-triazole; it has a different chemical structure to the imidazoles such as ketoconazole. It attacks the fungal cell wall causing leakage of cellular contents; it is water soluble and has a 30-hour half-life and this allows a single-dose regime.

Presentation
Capsules 150 mg.

Dose
One orally.

Contraindications
Pregnancy; lactation.

Indications
Vaginal candidiasis.

Side effects
Gastrointestinal upset.

Interactions
Anticoagulants; oral hypoglycaemics and phenytoin.

Special features
Single-dose regime for total body candidiasis.

Itraconazole

This is an oral broad-spectrum antifungal agent, highly active *in vitro* and *in vivo,* with a propensity to leave the bloodstream and achieve very high and persistent tissue levels.

Presentation

Capsules	100 mg.

Dose
Two capsules twice a day for 1 day.

Side effects
Nausea, abdominal pain, dyspepsia, headache.

Interactions
Rifampicin, cyclosporin, antacids, terfenadine, astemizole.

Ketoconazole

This is an imidazole-dioxolone antimycotic, effective after oral administration.

Presentation

Tablets	200 mg
Suspension	100 mg/5 ml
Cream	30 g, 2%

Dose
An oral dose of 200 mg twice a day for 5 days for *Candida albicans.* Apply cream twice daily.

Contraindications
Pregnancy; liver disease or abnormal liver-function tests.

Side effects
Nausea, rash, headache and pruritus have been observed. Hepatitis with an incidence of 1 in 10,000 patients has occurred. The hepatitis is reversible with cholestatic features; the drug should be stopped if jaundice occurs.

Special features
The tablets should always be taken with meals, since maximum absorption depends on stomach acidity. Drugs that reduce gastric secretions (anticholinergic drugs, antacids, H_2 blockers) should be taken at least 2 hours after ketoconazole. Interactions may also occur with phenytoin or anticoagulants.

Nystatin, BP, USP
This is an antifungal polyene antibiotic active against a wide range of yeasts and yeast-like fungi including *Candida albicans.* It acts on sterols in the fungal cell membrane to cause permeability and leakage of cell constituents.

Presentation

Cream	100,000 units/g
Gel	100,000 units/g
Pessaries	100,000 units/g
Tablets	500,000 units

Dose
Pessaries: One or two pessaries should be used vaginally for 15 consecutive nights regardless of any intervening menstrual period.
Cream: This should be applied three times a day and also every night. Support with nystatin oral tablets four times a day for 10 days or nystatin gel applied two-to-four times daily.

Contraindications
None known.

Indications
These include the treatment of vulvovaginal candidiasis.

Side effects
Occasional transient irritation and burning have been reported following insertion of the pessaries. Nausea, vomiting and diarrhoea may occur with nystatin tablets.

Special features
Oral preparations are listed and may be required to treat persistent and resistant gastrointestinal thrush. Nystatin is available as sugar-coated tablets for oral or

gastrointestinal moniliasis. In relapsing cases the treatment should be extended to ensure total eradication of all the fungal elements and all sources of re-infection. Recurrence rates after oral nystatin therapy are high. The USP preparation specifies not less than 4400 units/mg.

Amphotericin BP (Amphotericin B. USP) (see p. 8).

Local preparations

Local therapy with nystatin should preferably be continued for 6–10 days, but newer preparations are now available for single-dose use.

Clotrimazole

This has a broad spectrum of activity against fungi pathogenic to man. It is primarily fungistatic, but a fungicidal effect is achieved at concentrations in excess of 10–20 μg/ml. It is an imidazole derivative.

Presentation

Cream	1%, 2%, 10% VC
Vaginal tablets	100 mg, 200 mg, 500 mg

Dose

One 100 mg vaginal tablet should be used daily for 6 days, or one 200 mg vaginal tablet used daily for 3 days, or one 500 mg vaginal tablet as a single-dose treatment.

Contraindications

It should not be used during the menstrual period.

Indications

It is indicated for vulvovaginitis due to *Candida albicans.*

Side effects

Mild burning or irritation may arise.

Special features

Clotrimazole is also effective against infection by *Trichomonas vaginalis*, but systemic therapy with metronidazole is preferred for this condition. The 500 mg vaginal tablet is formulated with lactic acid to improve tissue penetration and release of the active ingredient. It has the advantage of a single application.

Econazole nitrate

This is an imidazole derivative.

Presentation

Cream	1% w/w
Pessaries	150 mg

Dose

Pessary: one inserted high into vagina at night as a single dose for 3 days.

Contraindications

Nil specific.

Side effects

Nil specific.

Special features

Econazole nitrate should not be used near the eyes.

Isoconazole nitrate

This is an imidazole derivative.

Presentation

Vaginal tablets 300 mg.

Dose

Two tablets inserted into the vagina as a single application.

Contraindications

Nil specific.

Side effects

Transient irritation and burning.

Special features

It has the advantage of a single application.

Miconazole nitrate

This is a phenethyl imidazole derivative similar to clotrimazole.

Presentation

Pessaries	100 mg
Cream	2%
Oral gel	2% w/w
Capsules	1200 mg

Dose

Cream: One full applicator of cream (5 g) should be used intravaginally at night for 14 days.

Pessaries: One pessary should be placed high into the vagina at night for 14 days.

Oral gel: 5–10 ml (miconazole 125–250 mg) four times daily.

Capsules: One inserted into vagina at night as a single dose.

Contraindications
None known.

Indications
It is indicated for the local treatment of vulvovaginal moniliasis.

Side effects
These include hypersensitivity, irritation and a burning sensation.

Special features
The cream, which should be stored in a cool place, can be used for the treatment of mycotic balanitis by applying to the affected area twice daily.

Miscellaneous
Other preparations occasionally used include:

Povidone-iodine (see p. 10).

Amphotericin, BP (amphotericin B, USP)
This, like nystatin, is a polyene antibiotic. The antifungal effects are maximal between pH 6.0 and 7.5 and decrease at low pH. It is nephrotoxic and in general is reserved for the treatment of visceral and septic mycoses in a hospital setting.

Presentation

Lozenges	10 mg	(10,000 units)
Suspension	100 mg/ml	(100,000 units)
Tablets	100 mg	(100,000 units)
Suspension 10% Cream Ointment Lotion 3%	for the treatment of candidiasis of skin and mucosae	

Dose
Oral preparations should be given four times daily for at least 14 days.

Contraindications
None known.

Indications
For the treatment of *Candida albicans* infection.

Side effects
No systemic or allergic reactions have been reported after local use. Anaphylaxis or renal impairment is common after parenteral use.

Special features
The drug is best reserved for parenteral use in systemic candidiasis and, if indicated, hospital admission will be required. It is now available where the drug is delivered in liposomes and is less toxic than conventional amphotericin B which is presented as a deoxycholate complex.

SUMMARY
After the eradication of predisposing factors, nystatin should be initially prescribed on cost grounds to treat *Candida albicans* infections. Failure to respond will indicate the need for newer imidazole derivatives. Oral itraconazole or fluconazole is indicated where there is recurrence of the infection or when local therapy is unacceptable.

Trichomonas vaginalis

This flagellated protozoan produces a greenish-yellow itchy discharge with an associated vaginitis and vulvitis. It is a transmissible venereal infection and all partners should be treated if abstinence from coitus is declined. It may be detected by cervical smear, cervical swabs or by examining a drop of discharge mixed with physiological saline, warmed to body temperature and under low-power magnification.

Systemic preparations

Metronidazole, BP, USP (see p. 39)
This systemic preparation is an imidazole derivative and is the established first-line treatment for *Trichomonas vaginalis* infections. It is also of proven value for prophylactic use in pelvic and abdominal surgery, since it is active against *Bacteroides* spp.

Presentation

Tablets	200 mg, 400 mg
Suppositories	500 mg, 1 g
Intravenous	500 mg in 100 ml infusion and 20 ml ampoule
Suspension	320 mg/5 ml benzoyl metronidazole (= 200 mg metronidazole)

Dose
An oral dose of 200 mg should be taken three times a day for 7 days, or 800 mg taken as a single dose in the morning and 1200 mg taken as a single dose at night for 2 days or 2 g as a strat dose.

Contraindications
There are no absolute contraindications, but the higher dosage regimens are not recommended in pregnancy or during lactation.

Indications
This is the treatment of choice for *Trichomonas vaginalis* infections, but metronidazole is also of value in other conditions including *Bacteroides* infections, amoebiasis, giardiasis, acute ulcerative gingivitis and dental infections and Bacterial vaginosis (see p. 12).

Side effects
Reported side effects include skin rashes or gastrointestinal disturbances, angioneuroma, central nervous system disturbances, dark urine, a furred tongue, leucopenia, urticaria, buccal ulceration and a metallic taste in the mouth. Neuropathy and epileptiform seizures may occur on long-term therapy.

Special features
The tablets should be swallowed, without chewing, with a half-glassful of water during or after meals. The suspension should be taken 1 hour before meals. Alcohol should be avoided, since interaction between alcohol and metronidazole leads to nausea and vomiting. Immediately pre-operatively and post-operatively, for the treatment of anaerobic infections, suppositories can be used. The intravenous preparations should preferably be reserved for more serious infections on cost grounds. Interactions can occur with alcohol, phenobarbitone or anticoagulants.

Local preparations

Povidone-iodine, USP
This vaginal preparation may be used for patients unable to tolerate oral preparations.

This is an iodine preparation and the active ingredient is water soluble, so the free iodine is slowly liberated. It is effective in the presence of pus, blood, serum and necrotic tissue and indications include candidiasis and trichomonal and non-specific vaginitis.

Presentation

Pessaries	200 mg
Vaginal gel	10% w/w
Douche	10% w/w

Dose

Pessaries: one pessary should be inserted into the vagina night and morning for 2–4 weeks.

Gel: a full applicator of gel (5 g) should be inserted into the vagina nightly for 2–4 weeks.

Douche: Two tablespoonfuls should be diluted in a pint of warm water and used as a vaginal douche daily (mornings usually).

Contraindications

Hypothyroidism.

Special features

Povidone-iodine pessaries are trichomonicidal and bactericidal and have been recommended for the pre-operative disinfection of the vagina. Povidone-iodine has also been used to treat herpes simplex and herpes zoster. It can cause both local skin reactions and allergic contact dermatitis and systemic adverse effects, if applied to denuded skin.

Chlamydia trachomatis

Chlamydial infection may be responsible for some cases of cervicitis and vaginitis. Tetracycline (see p. 36) or doxycycline are the antibiotics of choice or erythromycin (see p. 33) if tetracycline is contraindicated. Azithromycin dihydrate is also recommended.

Azithromycin (as dihydrate)

Presentation

Capsules	250 mg
Oral suspension	200 mg/5 ml

Dose

Four capsules as single dose.

Contraindications

Hepatic disease; pregnancy and lactation; renal impairment.

Side effects

Gastrointestinal upset; reversible elevation in liver enzymes; allergic reactions; rash; angioneurotic oedema; anaphylaxis.

Special features
Use with caution in renal or hepatic impairment, pregnancy or lactation. Interaction occurs with ergot derivatives, antacids or cyclosporin.

Bacterial vaginosis

Bacterial vaginosis was previously termed non specific vaginitis, Gardnerella vaginitis, Haemophilus vaginitis, Corynebacterium vaginitis and anaerobic vaginosis. Vaginosis appears to result from a change in vaginal ecology with the loss of normal lactobacilli and their replacement by a number of non-sporing anaerobes. Vaginosis can lead to serious problems including post-operative infection after hysterectomy, post-partum endometritis, premature rupture of membranes and pre-term delivery. A clinical diagnoses of Bacterial vaginosis is usually defined by a homogenous discharge and

1) ph greater than 4.5
2) positive amine test (vaginal secretions are alkalized and emit a "fishy" odour when mixed with 10% potassium hydroxide
3) Clue cells on microscopy.

The vagina cannot be sterilized, but local antisepsis may be obtained using topical agents.

Metronidazole gel (Not available in UK for Bacterial vaginosis) (see p .39)

Clindamycin Cream 2%
Use once daily for 7 days.

Both agents can be given systemically; metronidazole 200 mg three times a day for 7 days and clindamycin 300 mg twice daily for 7 days.

Sulphonamides
These may be considered for the treatment of non-specific bacterial vaginitis and cervicitis and for the prevention of bacterial infection after cervical surgery such as cautery to the cervix. The sulphonamides are not active against *Candida* or *Trichomonas* infections.

Presentation

Cream	Triple sulfa cream. sulphathiazole 3.42% w/w; sulphacetamide 2.86% w/w; sulphabenzamide 3.7% w/w (78 g tube).
Vaginal tablets	sulphathiazole 172.5 mg; sulphacetamide 143.75 mg sulphabenzamide 184 mg (20 vaginal tablets)

Dose
The cream should be applied to the affected areas and the vaginal tablets used twice daily for 10 days.

Special features
Sulphonamide sensitivity may occur.

> **SUMMARY**
> **The vagina can never be sterilized, but non-specific infections may be treated with local preparations. Vaginal douching is rarely recommended, since the normal vaginal acidity and bacterial flora may be disturbed.**

Genital herpes

This is associated with four features: increasing size of the problem, incurable and recurrent nature of the disease and neonatal infections and association with carcinoma of the cervix. Povidone-iodine (see p. 10) has been used for management. Acyclovir will reduce the duration of viral shedding and the duration of symptoms. It does not appear, however, to stop further recurrence.

Acyclovir

Presentation

Tablets	200 mg
Suspension	200 mg/5 ml
Cream 5% w/w	2 g, 10 g

Dose
An oral dose of 200 mg five times daily at 4-hourly intervals for 5 days or 5% w/w cream applied for a similar period.
For prophylaxis and suppression: 400 mg twice daily.

Contraindications
Hypersensitivity to acyclovir.

Side effects
Nil specific. Transient burning may follow application of the cream.

Special features
The dose should be reduced to 200 mg every 12 hours for patients with severe renal impairment. Interaction occurs with probenecid.

Gonorrhoea

Patients with proven gonorrhoea should be referred to the department of genito-urinary medicine for contact tracing and follow-up. Treatment regimens include:

1. Procaine penicillin 3.6 Mu/ml; probenecid 1 g as a single dose (see p. 24).
2. Ampicillin 2 g; probenecid 1 g as a single dose or Amoxycillin (see p. 24).
3. Acrosoxacin 300 mg as a single dose for patients who are allergic to penicillin or Ciprofloxacin (see p. 29); or Ofloxacin (see p. 29).
4. Spectinomycin — for males 1 g stat and for females 2 g (see p. 21).
5. Ceftriaxone 250 mg i.m. as a single dose (see p. 21).

Acrosoxacin

Presentation
Capsules 150 mg.

Dose
A single oral dose of 300 mg on an empty stomach.

Contraindications
Impaired renal or hepatic function.

Side effects
Dizziness, drowsiness, headaches, gastrointestinal disturbances. The patient's ability to drive or operate machinery may be impaired.

Special features
It is reserved for patients who are penicillin resistant or who have penicillin-resistant strains of gonorrhoea. It is not available in the United States.

Syphilis

Penicillin (see p. 24)
This remains the drug of choice.

Procaine penicillin, BP, USP

Presentation
Injection.

Dose
Intramuscular injection, 0.6–0.9 Mu, daily for 10 days.

Contraindications
Allergy to penicillin.

Side effects
Hypersensitivity reactions including pain and inflammatory reactions. Superinfections can result from changes in bacterial flora. Dermatitis and the Jarisch–Herxheimer skin reaction may occur.

Special features
For patients who are penicillin sensitive, erythromycin (see p. 33) or a cephalosporin (see p. 34) may be used.

Tuberculosis

This may be diagnosed at curettage during investigations for primary infertility; treatment should be in consultation with a consultant physician, but antituberculous agents are available, as described below.

Sodium aminosalicylate, BP, Eur.P, USP (PAS, *p*-aminosalicylic acid)
Benzoic and salicylic acids increase the oxygen consumption of the tubercle bacilli.

Presentation
Powder 100 g.

Dose
An oral dose of 8–12 g daily, in equally divided and spaced doses, reduced to 6–9 g daily when given simultaneously with isoniazid.

Contraindications
Salicylate hypersensitivity.

Side effects
Gastrointestinal tract irritation and peptic ulceration can occur. Hypersensitivity evident as fever, malaise, joint pains, skin eruption, neurological manifestations and impairment of hepatic function. Rarely, a syndrome resembling infectious mononucleosis can occur. Leucopenia, agranulocytosis or acute haemolytic anaemia may result. Allergic reactions can affect the lungs causing Loeffler's syndrome or perifocal infiltration. Liver and thyroid dysfunction and electrolyte disturbances, including acidosis and hypokalaemia, may also occur.

Special features
With impaired renal function, the dose should be reduced or salicylism can result. Aminosalicylic acid should be prescribed with either isoniazid, streptomycin or both.

Ethambutol hydrochloride, BP, USP
About 75% of human *Mycobacterium tuberculosis* strains are sensitive to 1 μg/ml of ethambutol. It inhibits the growth of *M. tuberculosis*. It is well absorbed with a long half-life.

Presentation
Tablets 100 mg, 400 mg.

Dose
An oral dose of 15 mg/kg daily as a single dose.

Contraindications
Nil specific.

Side effects
Dermatitis, pruritus and joint pains have been reported. The most important is optic neuritis, resulting in decrease of visual acuity, which is usually reversible on discontinuing the drug, and also loss of ability to perceive the colour green.

Special features
It is normally used in combination with other antituberculous therapy. Full visual tests should be performed. Caution is required with impaired renal function or during lactation.

Isoniazid BP, Eur.P, USP
This is the most important drug for the treatment of all types of tuberculosis; it is both tuberculostatic and tuberculocidal *in vivo*; the minimal tuberculostatic concentration is 0.025–0.05 mg/ml.

Presentation

Tablets	50 mg, 100 mg
Syrup	10 mg/ml
Injection	25 mg/ml

Dose
A total daily dose of 5 mg/kg with a maximum of 300 mg is given orally in two or three divided doses.

Contraindications
Nil specific.

Side effects
Hypersensitivity may present as skin eruptions, haematological reactions or arthritic symptoms. Peripheral neuritis, convulsions and optic neuritis followed by atrophy occasionally occur, as may hepatic damage. Other side effects include dryness of the mouth, epigastric distress, methaemoglobinaemia, tinnitus and pyridoxine deficiency anaemia.

Special features
The peripheral neuritis may be prevented by concurrent administration of pyridoxine. The human population shows genetic heterogeneity with regard to the rate of acetylation of isoniazid; there is a bimodal distribution. The variability is due to differences in the activity of an acetyl transferase. Patients who are slow inactivators may accumulate toxic concentrations if their renal

function is impaired and side effects include insomnia, restlessness, muscle twitching, psychotic disturbances, systemic lupus erythematosus-like symptoms and rheumatic syndrome.

Rifampicin BP (rifampin, USP)

This is highly active against *M. tuberculosis* but should always be used in combination with another drug.

Presentation

Capsules	150 mg, 300 mg
Syrup	100 mg/5 ml
Infusion	600 mg

Dose

A single oral dose of 600 mg daily or 8–12 mg/kg body weight.

Contraindications

Jaundice.

Side effects

Gastric intolerance and hypersensitivity, eosinophilia, leucopenia, hyperbilirubinaemia and a rise of plasma transaminases, fever, skin rashes and reddish discoloration of urine, sputum and tears.

Special features

As for all antituberculous drugs, rifampicin is used in combination with other antituberculous drugs. Interactions can occur with anticoagulants, corticosteroids, digitalis, hypoglycaemics, oral contraceptives, cyclosporin, dapsone, phenytoin, quinidine and narcotics.

Streptomycin sulphate, BP, Eur.P

Streptomycin sulphate has antibacterial activity against mycobacteria as well as many Gram-negative bacilli.

Presentation

Injection	1 g vial.

Dose

An intramuscular injection of 1 g per day (0.75 g daily for patients over 40 years).

Contraindications

Allergy to streptomycin and middle-ear diseases; particularly suppurative otitis media and labyrinthine disturbances.

Side effects
Skin sensitization may occur in persons handling the antibiotic, and rubber gloves are recommended. Ototoxicity with impairment of vestibular function, less often auditory function, can occur, particularly with prolonged therapy. A curare-like effect with apnoea and respiratory depression of motor and sensory neuropathy may occur following intraperitoneal application.

Special features
Sterile solutions of streptomycin sulphate should be used as soon as possible, but they can be kept for up to 28 days at less than 4°C. The injection should be given deeply into muscle and the site changed for each injection.

Pyrazinamide
This is an established component of many short course regimens. The combination of pyrazinamide with two or more antitubercular drugs is highly effective in killing mycobacteria. Hepatitis is minimized by keeping the daily dose to 30 mg/kg.

Presentation
Tablet 500 mg.

Dose
Maximum 3 g daily; 20–35 mg/kg daily in divided doses.

Special features
Monitor liver function and blood uric acid levels.

Atrophic vaginitis

This is normally treated using local or systemic oestrogen therapy (see p. 83) Alternative preparations available include acids aimed at restoring and maintaining vaginal acidity, since post-menopausally the vaginal pH is elevated from the normal pH 4.5 to that of a neutral or alkaline pH, with associated decreased resistance to infection. Such preparations include:

1. Lactic acid pessaries.
2. Dilute acetic acid jelly (Aci-Jel; Ortho).
3. Stilboestrol 0.5 mg and lactic acid 5% (Tampovagan; Norgine).

Contraindications
Oestrogens should not be used if there is a past history of carcinoma of the breast.

SUMMARY
Blind polypharmaceutical preparations are not advised. Treatment should be guided by the bacteriological sensitivities of cervical swabs. Predisposing factors, including diabetes mellitus, should be eliminated in patients with recurring infections.

Further reading

Easimon, C.S.F. (1993). The diagnosis and management of bacterial vaginosis. *Royal Society of Medicine Services Round Table Series* No. 30.

Feczk, J. (1989). Fluconazole; an overview if fluconazole and its role in vaginal candidiasis, *International Congress and Symposium Series* 160 (ed. R.G. Richardson). Royal Society of Medicine Services, London, New York.

Hillier, S.L. (1992). Clindamycin treatment of bacterial vaginosis. *Reviews Contemporary Pharmacotherapy*, No. 3, 263–268.

Kinghorn, G.R. (1989). Vaginal candidiasis: an overview. pp1–6 In "Fluconazole and its role in Vaginal candidiasis" Royal Society Syndicate Services Ltd No 160

Leading article (1992). Chlamydial infections. *Therapeutic Options*, **339,** 711–713.

Magee, P. (1993). Adverse reactions; povidone-iodine; *Prescribers Journal*, **33**(4). 160–163.

Stewart, J.C.M., Ferguson J. and Davey, P. (1983). New antifungal and antiviral chemotherapy. *British Medical Journal*, **286**, 1802.

Sobel, J.D. (1990) Vaginal Infections in Adult Women, *Sexually Transmitted Diseases* **74**(6), 1573–1602.

Chapter 2

Infections

Introduction

Therapeutic measures other than antibiotics alone are of importance in the management of acute or chronic pelvic inflammatory disease and include intravenous fluids, diet, rest, nursing care, psychotherapy, physiotherapy and surgery.

Specific antibacterial agents (see Table 2.1) are indicated in the management of urinary-tract infections, intra-amniotic infections, pelvic inflammatory disease, including septicaemia and septic abortions, and breast abscesses.

A liberal fluid intake is advised for high fever and urinary tract infections and the value of aspirin as an antipyretic agent should be remembered. The development of *Candida albicans* infection following antibiotic use may require appropriate therapy (see Chapter l).

Prophylaxis

Prophylactic antibiotics (penicillin, amoxycillin or cephalosporin) to prevent subacute bacterial endocarditis should be given to cardiac patients with stenotic lesions undergoing surgery, while metronidazole is used prophylactically against anaerobic infections prior to pelvic surgery and sulfametopyrazine may be given prophylactically against urinary-tract infections when catheterization is planned. Antibiotics (especially Amoxycillin and clavulanic acid or a cephalosporin) are also given prophylactically prior to pelvic surgery, including vaginal repair and hysterectomy. Many hospitals have Drug and Therapeutics committees and devise local Manuals of Antibiotic Practice, and practitioners should always contact the local Department of Microbiology if any particular problems arise.

Cefoxitin (as sodium salt)

This is but *one* example of an antibiotic used for pre-operative prophylaxis.

Dose

2 g i.m. or i.v., 30 minutes to 1 hour pre-operatively, then 6-hourly for 24 hours. For caesarean sections 2 g i.v. is given on clamping the cord.

Table 2.1 Antibiotics and antibacterials (Not all are listed in the text and many others are marketed at intervals)

Aminoglycosides
Amikacin
Gentamicin
Kanamycin
Neomycin
Netilmicin
Spectinomycin
Tobramycin

Carbapenems
Imipenem

Cephalosporins
Cefaclor
Cefadroxil
Cefamandole
Cefixime
Cefodizime*
Cefotaxime
Cefoxitin
Cefpodoxime
Cefsulodin*
Ceftibuten
Cefuroxime
Ceftriaxone
Cephadoxione*
Cephalexin
Cephazolin
Cephradine

Folic acid inhibitors
Trimethoprim

Fusicid Acid
Fusidic Acid

Hexamine derivatives
Hexamine hippurate
Hexamine mandelate

Lincosamide
Clinadmycin

Macrolides
Azithromycin
Clarithromycin
Erythromycin (and salts)

Nitrofurans
Nitrofurantoin

Nitroimidazoles
Metronidazole
Tinidazole

Penicillins
Broad spectrum
- Amoxycillin
- Ampicillin
- Bacampicillin*
- Piperacillin
- Pivampicillin*
- Talampicillin*

Penicillinase sensitive
- Benzathine penicillin
- Penicillin G
- Penicillin G + procaine penicillin
- Penicillin G + procaine penicillin G + benethamine penicillin G
- Penicillin V

Penicillinase resistant
- Cloxacillin
- Flucloxacillin*
- Methicillin
- Temocillin*

Antipseudomonal penicillins
- Axiocillin*
- Carbenicillin
- Micarcillin*

Amidinopenicillins
- Mecillinam*
- Pivmecillinam*

Combinations
- Ampicillin + cloxacillin
- Ampicillin + flucloxacillin
- Ampicillin + sulbactam
- Amoxycillin + clavulanic acid
- Pivampicillin + pivmecillinam
- Ticarcillin + clavulanic acid

Phosphoric Acid Derivative
Fosfomycin

Quinolones
Acrosoxacin*
Cinoxacin*
Ciprofloxacin
Nalidixic acid
Norfloxacin
Ofloxacin

Sulphonamides
Sulfametopyrazine

Combinations
- Trimethoprim + sulphamethoxazole

Tetracyclines
Chlortetracycline
Demeclocycline*
Doxycycline
Lymecycline*
Minocycline
Oxytetracycline
Tetracycline

Combinations
- Tetracycline + nystatin
- Tetracycline + chlortetracycline + demeclocycline

* Not available in the United States

Contraindications
Penicillin sensitivity, renal insufficiency.

Side effects
Gastrointestinal disturbance, eosinophilia, neutropenia, leucopenia, thrombocytopenia, rise in liver enzymes and blood urea, positive Coombs test.

Special features
Interaction can occur with loop diuretics and aminoglycosides.

Urinary-tract infections

Normally, a short course of antibiotic (3–5 days) will clear any infection but occasionally, where there is underlying renal pathology, long-term therapy is required. Suitable drugs for urinary-tract infections include trimethoprim, penicillins, quinolones, the cephalosporins (see p. 30), noxythiolin, hexamine derivatives. Fosfomycin trometamol is a new agent licensed as a single dose treatment for acute uncomplicated urinary-tract infections.

Sulphonamides

Co-trimoxazole (trimethoprim, BP; sulphamethoxazole, BP)
This contains trimethoprim 80 mg (see p. 23) and sulphamethoxazole 400 mg. The objective of therapy with trimethoprim-sulphamethoxazole is the depletion of the microbial tetrahydrofolate (an essential catalyst for the biosynthesis of constituents of nucleic acids and coenzymes and serine) to levels incompatible with function and life. This is accomplished by the selective inhibition of the microbial dihydrofolate reductase by trimethoprim, together with the inhibition of the biosyntheses of dihydrofolate by sulphamethoxazole.

Presentation

Dispersible tablets	(single and double strength)
Dispersible capsules	(single and double strength)
Suspension	one tablet = 5 ml suspension
Injection	5 ml i.m., 5 ml infusion

Dose

Tablets/capsules	one to three should be taken twice daily for 10–14 days
Suspension	5–15 ml twice daily

Contraindications
These include pregnancy and severe renal insufficiency, liver parenchymal damage, blood dyscrasias and patients with sulphonamide sensitivity.

Side effects

Those reported include nausea and vomiting, glossitus, skin rashes, blood changes including thrombocytopenia, purpura, leucopenia, neutropenia and, rarely, agranulocytosis, erythema multiforme, Lyell syndrome.

Special features

Trimethoprim may be prescribed as a single ingredient, but resistant strains to trimethoprim are now developing. Interaction can occur with folate inhibitors, anticoagulants, anticonvulsants and hypoglycaemia.

Trimethoprim, BP

This is a folic acid inhibitor and not a sulphonamide, but is included in this section for completeness.

Presentation

Tablets	100 mg, 200 mg
Suspension	50 mg/5 ml

Dose

Therapeutic, 200 mg twice a day; long-term or prophylactic, 100 mg at night.

Contraindications

(See co-trimoxazole)

Side effects

See co-trimoxazole.

Special precautions

(See co-trimoxazole)

Sulfametopyrazine

Catheterization of the urethra and bladder increases the risk of urinary-tract infection and long-acting sulphonamides may be given pre-operatively to patients undergoing gynaecological surgery or where post-operative long-term catheterization is required. Unfortunately, the majority of *Escherichia coli* organisms, commonly the cause of urinary-tract infections, are now sulphonamide resistant. Urine cultures are therefore indicated.

Presentation

Tablets 2 g.

Dose

An oral dose of 2 g should be taken once weekly. The tablet should be stirred into a half-tumblerful of water or orange squash. The suspension may be diluted with syrup.

Contraindications
These include pregnancy and sulphonamide hypersensitivity.

Side effects
These are as for all sulphonamides (see p. 22).

Special features
The long half-life of sulfametopyrazine is due to a high degree of renal tubular re-absorption coupled with a low rate of hepatic metabolism of the drug. If elimination of the drug is required, the urine should be made alkaline (pH 8) by means of potassium citrate mixture.

Penicillins

Compounds from this large group all act as inhibitors of bacterial cell-wall synthesis. Molecular modifications are marketed at regular intervals and examples include finidazole, mecillinam hydrochloride, mezlocillin and ticarcillin sodium. They should only be prescribed after consultation with the local consultant microbiologist.

Amoxycillin trihydrate, BP
This is the penicillin of choice and is better absorbed than ampicillin. Probenecid, which blocks renal tubular excretion, may be used to increase blood levels of penicillins, but it is not indicated for mild urinary-tract infections. In combination with clavulinic acid (Augmentin; Beecham) (see below), it may be used as a substitute for both ampicillin/probenecid and metronidazole in pelvic inflammatory disease. It is also used to treat gonorrhoea and prophylactically to prevent endocarditis.

Presentation

Capsules	250 mg, 500 mg
Syrup	250 mg/5 ml
Injections	250 mg/5 ml; 500 mg; 1 g
Sachets	3 g

Dose

Urinary tract infection:	3 g repeated once 12 hours later.
Gonorrhoea:	3 g single dose.
Pelvic inflammatory disease:	500 mg t.d.s.; in severe infections 500 mg i.m. 8-hourly or 1 g i.v. 6-hourly.
Prophylaxis of endocarditis:	1 g single dose pre-surgery; 500 mg orally 6 hours later.

Contraindications
Known penicillin hypersensitivity.

Side effects
Mild cases of diarrhoea, indigestion and erythematous rash have been reported.

Special features
A single 3 g dose may cure uncomplicated infections. However, amoxycillin trihydrate is similar to benzylpenicillin G and phenoxymethylpenicillin (penicillin V) in that it is destroyed by bacterial β-lactamases so that staphylococci which produce β-lactamase are resistant. Other penicillins are marketed, but these especially should only be prescribed when bacteriological sensitivities are available.

Amoxycillin with clavulanic acid (Augmentin)
Resistance to many antibiotics is caused by bacterial enzymes which destroy the antibiotic before it can act on the pathogen. The clavulanate anticipates this defence mechanism by blocking the β-lactamase enzymes, thus rendering the organisms sensitive to amoxycillin's rapid bactericidal effect at concentrations readily attainable in the body. Clavulanate by itself has little antibacterial activity; however, in association with amoxycillin, it produces an antibiotic agent of broad spectrum with wide application in hospital and general practice.

The pharmacokinetics of the two components of Augmentin are closely matched. Peak serum levels of both occur about 1 hour after oral administration. Both clavulanate and amoxycillin have low levels of serum binding; about 70% remains free in the serum.

Presentation

Tablets	Amoxycillin trihydrate plus potassium clavulanate 375 mg, 625 mg
Dispersible tablets	375 mg
Suspension	100 ml, (250/62 / 5 ml) (125/31 / 5 ml)

Dose
375 mg t.d.s. or 625 mg t.d.s. for severe infection. If there is moderate renal impairment, reduce dose to 12-hourly regime. If there is severe renal impairment reduce dose to 375 mg b.d.

Side effects
Prolongation of bleeding time and prothrombin time have been reported in some patients; care should be used in patients on anticoagulation therapy. Changes in liver-function tests can occur and care should be used in patients with severe hepatic dysfunction. Cholestatic jaundice (reversible) has been rarely reported. It can occur up to 6 weeks after stopping therapy. Urticarial

and erythematous rashes, angio-oedema and anaphylaxis have all been reported.

Special features

The dose should be reduced (see above) in patients with renal impairment.

Nitrofurans

Nitrofurantoin, BP

This is a synthetic nitrofuran and acts by interfering with bacterial DNA. Its antibacterial activity is greater at acidic urine. It is bactericidal to most Gram-positive and Gram-negative urinary-tract pathogens (except *Pseudomonas aeruginosa*) in renal tissue and throughout the urinary tract. After oral administration, nitrofurantoin is rapidly excreted in the urine, with up to 45% being unchanged.

Presentation

Tablets	50 mg, 100 mg
Suspension	25 mg/5 ml

Dose

Divided doses 400 mg (100 mg four times a day) should be taken daily, with food.

Long-term suppression 50–100 mg once daily at night.

Prophylaxis 50 mg four times daily during procedure and 3 days after.

Contraindications

These include anuria or marked oliguria and glucose-6-phosphate dehydrogenase deficiency.

Indications

It may be used for the treatment of urinary-tract infection in pregnancy except at term.

Side effects

Haemolysis may occur in patients with glucose-6-phosphate dehydrogenase deficiency in their erythrocytes. Other side effects include nausea and vomiting, peripheral neuropathy, drug rashes and pyrexia. Bronchospasm and/or dyspnoea, cough and chest pain have also been reported, but are very rare. These symptoms may be associated with transitory pulmonary infiltration or pleural effusion. Liver-function tests may be disordered.

Special features

It is also available as macrocrystalline nitrofuran. The tablets should be taken with food and milk to minimize the incidence of nausea and vomiting.

Interaction can occur with magnesium trisilicate, probenecid, sulphinpyrazone and the quinolones.

Quinolones

Quinolones are bactericidal and act by inhibiting the enzyme responsible for supercoiling the DNA strands during bacterial replication. They provide effective bactericidal activity against a wide range of Gram-negative bacteria but are less effective against Gram-positive bacteria.

Nalidixic acid

This is recommended for acute and chronic infections caused by Gram-negative pathogens other than *Pseudomonas* spp.

Presentation

Suspension	300 mg/5 ml
Tablets	500 mg
Sachets	660 mg

Dose

An oral dose of 1 g should be taken four times daily (it may be reduced to 2 g daily for long-term therapy), or 15 ml four times a day for 7 days.

Contraindications

It should be used with caution in patients in the first trimester of pregnancy and in patients with liver disease and where there is a history of convulsive disorders. Patients should avoid excessive exposure to sunlight.

Side effects

These include gastrointestinal effects and skin reactions or subjective visual disturbances may occur. There are also isolated reports of convulsive episodes (usually associated with overdosage). A haemolytic reaction may be precipitated in glucose-6-phosphate-deficient individuals. Interaction occurs with probenecid and anticoagulants.

Special features

There is no parenteral preparation available. Nalidixic acid may interfere with the estimation of urinary ketosteroids and urinary vanilmandelic acid. Clinistix (Ames) or Tes-Tape (Lilly) should be used for urinary sugar determination, since other methods may give false positive results. If given to patients on anticoagulation therapy, the dose of anticoagulant may have to be reduced.

Citrated nalidixic acid sachets

These contain nalidixic acid 660 mg.

Dose
One sachet three times a day for 3 days.

Special features
Sodium citrate included in the formulation of the sachet raises the urinary pH. This causes the amount of free nalidixic acid and active metabolites in the urine to more than double as a result of a corresponding reduction in inactive glucuronides.

Norfloxacin
This is a more potent derivative of nalidixic acid.

Presentation
Tablets 400 mg.

Dose
One tablet twice a day for 3–10 days; for chronic urinary-tract infections one tablet twice a day for 12 weeks.

Contraindications
Pregnancy, lactation, growing adolescents.

Side effects
Nausea, headache, dizziness, rash, heartburn, abdominal cramp, diarrhoea, anorexia, sleep disturbances, anxiety, irritability, convulsions. It should be used with caution with a history of renal impairment or epilepsy.

Special features
Interaction occurs with nitrofurantoin, theophylline, cyclosporin, oral anticoagulants, sucralfate, antacids, probenecid and non-steroidal anti-inflammatory drugs.

Cinoxacin
This quinolone is indicated for urinary-tract infection.

Presentation
Capsules 500 mg.

Dose
One, twice daily for 7–14 days.
Prophylactically one at night.

Contraindications
As norfloxacin.

Side effects
As norfloxacin.

Special features
As norfloxacin.

Ciprofloxacin (hydrochloride; monohydrate)
This 4-quinolone is active against a wide range of both Gram-negative and Gram-positive organisms including those resistant to penicillins, cephalosporins or aminoglycosides.

Presentation

Tablets	100 mg, 500 mg
Infusion	2 mg/ml

Dose
250–750 mg twice daily.

Gonorrhoea:	250 mg single dose
Severe infections:	750 mg twice daily

Contraindications
Pregnancy; lactation; use with caution with epilepsy, history of CNS disorders; patients should be well hydrated; patients with glucose-6-phosphate defects; driving or operating machinery.

Side effects
Local irritation; pain at infection site; gastrointestinal disturbance; dizziness; headache; tremor; confusion; convulsions; rashes; blurred vision; joint pain; impaired judgement; transient increases in serum creatinine. Haematological hepatic disturbances; vasculitis; pseudomembranous colitis; Stevens–Johnson syndrome; tachycardia.

Special features
Interacts with theophylline (monitor plasma levels); cyclosporin (monitor serum creatinine); magnesium, aluminium or iron salts; alcohol; anticoagulants; non-steroidal anti-inflammatory drugs.

Ofloxacin
This is a 4-quinolone.

Presentation

Tablets	200 mg.

Dose
Two once daily in morning for 5–10 days.

Gonorrhoea:	two as a single dose.

Contraindications
History of epilepsy; pregnancy; lactation.

Side effects
Gastrointestinal upset; hypersensitivity; skin reactions; convulsions; CNS disturbances; pseudomembranous colitis; transient increases in liver enzymes; rarely joint muscle pain; bone-marrow depression.

Special features
Interacts with magnesium.

Acrosoxacin (see p. 14)
This 4-quinolone is specifically indicated for acute gonorrhoea; 2g capsules are given as a single dose.

> **NOTE:**
> A quinolone antibiotic — temafloxacin — has caused serious and fatal adverse reactions including haemolytic anaemia, hypoglycaemia, renal failure, hepatic dysfunction and anaphylaxis. Similar adverse reactions have been reported with other quinolones but in much lower frequency and continued pharmacovigilance is indicated.

Cephalosporins (see p. 34)

Most cephalosporins are used in pelvic inflammatory disease (see p. 33); however ceftibuten dihydrate is available as a 400mg single dose regime for urinary tract infection.

Fosfomycin trometamol

Fosfomycin trometamol is a broad-spectrum antibiotic with activity against the major urinary-tract pathogens. It contains the trometamol salt of fosfomycin, a phosphonic acid derivative antibiotic produced by the bacterium *Streptomyces fradiae*. Fosfomycin is a bactericidal agent which inhibits bacterial cell-wall synthesis. It inactivates the enzyme pyruvyltransferase, which is responsible for the condensation of phosphoenolpyruvate with UDP-N-acetylglucosamine in the formation of UDP-N-acetylmuramic acid. This is the first step in the synthesis of peptidoglycan, a component of almost all bacterial cell walls. Without the ability to produce peptidoglycan, the bacteria are unable to survive.

It has a broad spectrum of activity and at concentrations reached in urine is active against most Gram-positive and Gram-negative organisms involved in urinary-tract infections.

Dose
3g single dose for urinary tract infection; for prophylaxis 3g pre procedure and repeat after 24 hours.

Contraindications
Severe renal impairment.

Side effects
Gastrointestinal disturbance.

Special features
Interacts with metoclopramide

Hexamine derivatives

Hexamine hippurate (methenamine hippurate) and hexamine mandelate (Methenamine mandelate, USP)

These are urinary antibacterial agents with a twofold antibacterial action — the slow release of the bactericidal formaldehyde and the bacteriostatic effect of hippuric acid. They should be reserved for chronic urinary-tract infections or for patients with indwelling catheters.

Presentation

Tablets	hexamine mandelate	250 mg, 500 mg
	hexamine hippurate	1 g

Dose
Hexamine hippurate: an oral dose of 1 g twice daily. Hexamine mandelate: 1g, 6-hourly.

Indications
They are indicated on a prophylactic basis against the introduction of infection into the urinary tract during instrumental procedures and to suppress urinary infections in patients with indwelling catheters. They are also used for long-term therapy in the prevention of recurrent cystitis.

Contraindications
They should not be used concurrently with sulphonamides because of the possibility of crystalluria, or with alkalizing agents such as potassium citrate mixture. They are also contraindicated in patients with hepatic insufficiency, severe dehydration, metabolic acidosis or severe renal failure.

Side effects
These include rashes, gastric irritation and bladder irritation.

Special features
Should be taken in the presence of acidified urine for maximum effect.

Bladder antiseptics

For patients with indwelling catheters, bladder irrigations using noxythiolin may also be considered. It is a urinary antiseptic. Mandelic acid 1% solutions are also available for the prevention or reduction of infection with indwelling catheters.

Noxythiolin

Presentation
Powder 2.5 g.

Dose
By irrigation, 1–2.5% solution.

Side effects
A burning sensation may be noticed.

Special features
It is also available with amethocaine hydrochloride. A similar preparation containing local anaesthetic, chlorhexidine gluconate and methyl- and propylhydroxybenzoate is also available.

Intra-amniotic infections

Ruptured membranes alone do not necessarily indicate the need for an antibiotic, since long-term therapy will lead to tolerance to the antibiotic and other parameters such as pyrexia, and positive bacterial cultures from cervical swabs should be available prior to prescribing antibiotics.

Intra-amniotic infection may, however, be present without symptoms, but convincing evidence is lacking that systemic prophylactic therapy helps. After 34–36 weeks' gestation, the risk of neonatal pneumonia is higher than the risk of prematurity and the infant should be delivered, preferably by the vaginal route. If the infant has died, a vaginal delivery should be arranged and antibiotic cover provided.

Parenteral ampicillin, a cephalosporin, or clindamycin hydrochloride are advised pending bacteriological sensitivity.

Amoxycillin trihydrate, BP (see p. 24)
The parent compound, ampicillin, has been shown to cross the placental barrier. Oral amoxycillin should be prescribed initially, but parenteral ampicillin will be required in labour.

Cephalosporins (see p. 34)
These have a broad spectrum of activity and are of value for intra-amniotic infection, urinary-tract infections and pelvic inflammatory disease.

Clindamycin hydrochloride, USP (see p 37)
The parent compound, lincomycin, was previously used for the treatment of amnionitis, but clindamycin is now advised, being better absorbed and unaffected by food. It is active against infections caused by staphylococci, pneumococci, streptococci (other than enterococci) and anaerobic infections caused by organisms such as *Bacteroides* spp. It is best used in the management of patients with pelvic inflammatory disease, but pseudomembranes colitis if used for more than a few days may occur. It is also recommended in the management of Bacterial Vaginosis (p. 121).

Pelvic inflammatory disease

Antibiotics are normally prescribed in the acute or chronic phase of pelvic inflammatory disease, but anti-inflammatory drugs are also of value in chronic disease. Antibiotics are used in the management of septic abortion and should be given intravenously at least 12 hours prior to curettage and post-operatively for 5–7 days; Gram-negative septicaemic shock may occur.

For non-gonococcal pelvic infection, the alternative antibiotics include the following:

Penicillins

Amoxycillin trihydrate, BP (see p. 24)
This is a broad-spectrum antibiotic active against Gram-positive organisms including penicillin-sensitive *Staphylococcus aureus, Streptococcus pyogenes, S. faecalis and S. viridans*, and also Gram-negative organisms including *Escherischia coli* and *Proteus mirabilis*. It is also active against *Neisseria gonorrhoea*.

Flucloxacillin sodium (see p. 41)
This is indicated for infections due to Gram-positive organisms including penicillin-resistant staphylococci. It is best reserved for treating breast abscess due to *Staphylococcus aureus*.

Macrolides

This group includes erythromycin, azithromycin, clarithromycin and spiramycin. Azithromycin and clarithromycin (which is used for respiratory tract infections and skin and soft tissue infections) cause fewer side effects than erythromycin. Spiramycin is used against toxoplasmosis on a named patient basis.

Erythromycin, BP, Eur.P, USP

This is useful as a penicillin substitute in allergic patients, since it has a good spectrum of activity against Gram-positive organisms such as staphylococci and it is also effective against most anaerobes including *Bacteroides fragilis*. It is also used for the treatment of *Chlamydia trachomatis* infection.

Presentation

Capsules	erythromycin estolate 125 mg, 250 mg
Oral suspension	erythromycin estolate 25 mg/ml, 50 mg/ml, 100 mg/ml
Tablets	erythromycin estolate 125 mg, 250 mg, 500 mg
Injection	erythromcyin lactobionate 0.5 g, 1 g

Dose

Divided doses, 1–2 g daily, for up to 10 days orally or by intravenous infusion.

Contraindications

Impaired liver function and previous hypersensitivity to erythromycin.

Side effects

Liver dysfunction; patients with hepatic dysfunction should not receive the estolate; hypersensitivity reaction (fever, eosinophilia and skin eruption); gastrointestinal irritation (epigastric distress); thrombophlebitis after intravenous injections.

Special features

Erythromycin gluceptate is mainly used in the United States — it is very similar to erythromycin lactobionate. Erythromycin stearate is also available — it can be given twice a day and better blood levels can be obtained.

Azithromycin (see p. 11)

This macrolide is active against *Chlamydia trachomatis*.

Presentation

Capsules 250 mg.

Dose

Two, once daily for 3 days, 2 hours before meals, or two as a single dose on day 1 and one daily for next 4 days.

Genital infection: four as a single dose.

Contraindications

Pregnancy; renal impairment.

Side effects
Gastrointestinal upset; reversible elevation of liver enzymes. Interacts with ergot derivatives, antacids and cyclosporin.

Cephalosporins

These are recommended for septicaemia due to *Staphylococcus aureus, Proteus mirabilis, Escherichia coli* and *Klebsiella* spp.

First and second generation

Presentation
Oral:
(a) Cephradine
  Capsules 250 mg, 500 mg
  Suspension 125 mg/5 ml, 250 mg/5 ml
(b) Cephalexin, BP, USP
  Tablets 500 mg, 250 mg
  Capsules 500 mg, 250 mg
  Suspension 125 mg/5 ml, 250 mg/5 ml
Parenteral:
(a) Cephradine
  Injection 500 mg, 1 g

Dose
Parenteral: 2–4 g should be given every 6 hours, either by intramuscular injection or by intravenous infusion.
Oral: 250 mg–500 g every 6 hours.

Third generation (cefuroxime sodium)

This third-generation cephalosporin has a substantial resistance to β-lactamase enzymes produced by many Gram-negative organisms. It is bactericidal in

Table 2.2 Oral cephalosporins:

Drug	Suggested regimen (adults) as doses per day
Cefaclor	250–500 mg three times
Cefadroxil	0.5–1.0 g two times
Cefixime	200 mg twice or 400 mg once
Cefpodoxime	100–200 mg two times
Cefuroxime	250–500 mg two times
Cephalexin	250 mg four times or 500 mg three times
Cephradine	250–500 mg four times

action and inactivates transpeptidase enzymes involved in bacterial cell-wall biosynthesis.

Presentation
Injection 250 mg, 750 mg, 1.5 g.

Dose
Intramuscular or intravenous injection, 500–750 mg 3 times daily, increased to 1–2 g three times daily for very severe infections.

Contraindications
These include hypersensitivity to cephalosporins and concomitant therapy with diuretics, since renal failure has occurred with the combination of cephalosporins and diuretic therapy.

Side effects
Although usually well tolerated by patients who are penicillin allergic, cross-reaction has been encountered. Nausea, vomiting, diarrhoea and, as with other broad-spectrum antibiotics, overgrowth with commensal organisms such as *Candida* spp. can occur during oral therapy. Rare cases of neutropenia and skin rashes have been reported.

Special features
They may be given to patients who are allergic to penicillin, noting the potential for cross-reaction.

SUMMARY
Cephaloridine and cephalothin sodium have similar antibacterial activities against most bacteria. Cephalexin and cephradine have a lower antibacterial activity against Gram-positive bacteria than cephaloridine or cephalothin sodium. Cefuroxime sodium has a high degree of resistance to many β-lactamase enzymes from Gram-negative organisms and is active against hospital strains of *Klebsiella* and *Escherichia coli*. Newer cephalosporins are becoming available and consultation with the local consultant microbiologist is advisable.

Sulphonamides

These are recommended against *Escherichia coli* and *Proteus* spp.

Co-trimoxazole (see p. 22)

Tetracyclines

There are many — this group includes:

Tetracycline hydrochloride
Doxycycline
Chlortetracycline
Oxytetracycline
Minocycline
Lymecycline
Demeclocycline

They are all recommended for pelvic inflammatory disease and show common features.

Tetracycline hydrochloride, BP, Eur.P, USP
This is active against *Chlamydia* and *Mycoplasma* spp.

Presentation

Tablets	250 mg
Injection	100 mg, 250 mg, 500 mg

Dose
250–500 mg q.i.d.
100 mg i.m. two to three times daily or 500 mg 12-hourly by i.v. infusion.

Contraindications
Pregnancy, lactation, systemic lupus erythematosus, intracranial hypertension.

Side effects
Gastrointestinal disturbances, allergic reactions, superinfections, intracranial hypertension.

Special features
Use cautiously with renal or hepatic impairment; interacts with milk, antacids, mineral supplements and oral contraceptives.

Lincosamide

Clindamycin hydrochloride
This is a member of the lincosamides group of agents based on a novel structure unlike that of any other antibiotic. It is active against Gram-positive organisms and also some anaerobic and Gram-negative organisms including *Bacteroides* spp. It is not active against *Streptococcus faecalis.*

Presentation

Capsules	75 mg, 150 mg
Injection (as phosphate)	150 mg/ml

Dose
150–450 mg 6-hourly
600mg–2.7 g by i.m. injection or i.v. infusion daily in divided doses.

Contraindications
Lincomycin sensitivities; colitis.

Side effects
Pseudomembranous colitis; jaundice or blood disorders.

Special features
Use cautiously with renal or hepatic impairment; interacts with neuromuscular blocking agents.

Aminoglycosides

Gentamicin sulphate, BP, USP
This is active against Gram-positive and Gram-negative pathogens including *Escherichia coli*, *Klebsiella* spp., *Proteus* spp., *Pseudomonas aeruginosa* and *Staphylococcus aureus*. It is an aminoglycoside. Other members of this group of drugs include streptomycin, kanamycin (see below), neomycin and the newer aminoglycosides, tobramycin and amikacin. All drugs exhibit a moderate toxicity and should be strictly monitored. Neomycin is reserved for oral use in the context of reducing gastrointestinal flora pre-operatively, but others are used parenterally.

Presentation
Injection 2 ml = 80 mg gentamicin base.

Dose
For 60 kg body weight or over, 80 mg should be given every 8 hours either intramuscularly or intravenously for 7–10 days; for less than 60 kg body weight, 60 mg should be given every 8 hours either intramuscularly or intravenously for 7–10 days. For serious systemic infections, 5 mg/kg body weight may be given in equally divided doses at 6- or 8-hourly intervals.

Contraindications
These include pregnancy (except in life-threatening situations). Patients who have had an earlier course of gentamicin sulphate, or who are receiving any other aminoglycoside antibiotic, frusemide or other potentially nephrotoxic or ototoxic drug, should be treated with alternative antibiotics whenever possible. If this is not possible, strict monitoring of serum levels should be maintained, avoiding levels of above 10 μg/ml.

Side effects

Patients with renal impairment are more liable to ototoxicity from exposure to gentamicin sulphate. Other side effects include nephrotoxicity and allergic reactions.

Special features

Blood levels should be monitored and liaison with the local Department of Microbiology is advised. The best guide to dosage schedules in adults is the nomogram designed by Mawer *et al.* (1974).

Kanamycin sulphate, BP, USP

This is advised for the treatment of Gram-negative organisms resistant to other antibiotics.

Presentation

Injection 4 ml, 250 mg/ml.

Dose

For acute infections: 1 g daily should be given by intramuscular injection in two-to-four divided doses; not more than 10 g should be given. For chronic infections, 1 g on alternate days should be given by intramuscular injection in divided doses; not more than 50 g should be given.

Kanamycin sulphate may be given intravenously for gravely ill patients with overwhelming infections or with impending vascular collapse. It may be given by slow intravenous infusion (2.5 mg/ml at 3–4 ml per minute), providing a dose of 15–30 mg/kg body weight daily in two or three divided doses.

Contraindications

Nil specific.

Side effects

Reported side effects include the following: intolerance to intramuscular injection, ecchymoses and sensitivity rashes; a curare-like effect with apnoea and respiratory depression or motor and sensory neuropathy has been noticed following intraperitoneal application; tinnitus and loss of hearing (which may be permanent) and hyaline granular urinary casts may also be observed.

Special features

The drug is best reserved for seriously ill patients, and blood antibiotic levels should be monitored to prevent a rise above 30 μg/ml.

Nitroimidazoles

Metronidazole, BP, USP (see p. 9)

This is recommended for *Bacteroides* spp. (especially *B. fragilis*), and also fusobacteria, eubacteria, clostridia and anaerobic streptococci. It is advised in preventing or treating post-operative infections by killing the most important obligate anaerobic bacteria. It is recommended after surgery involving the lower bowel or pelvic organs.

This is also recommended for the treatment of trichomonal vaginal infections (see p. 9) and for anaerobic sepsis due to *Bacteroides* spp. or anaerobic streptococci.

Presentation

Tablets	200 mg, 400 mg
Suspension	320 mg/5 ml = metronidazole 200 mg (benzoyl metronidazole)
Suppositories	500 mg, 1 g
Injection	500 mg/100 ml (for intravenous infusion)

Dose
Initially 800 mg and then 400 mg tablets should be taken three times a day during or after meals for a minimum of 7 days. For prophylaxis in gynaecological surgery, a single oral dose of 2 g should be given on admission, followed by 200 mg three times a day until pre-operative starvation is started. Post-operatively, 200 mg should be given three times a day for 7 days.

Contraindications
There are no absolute contraindications. Care should be taken with hepatic encephalopathy and CNS disorders.

Side effects
Those reported include unpleasant taste in the mouth, furred tongue, nausea and vomiting and buccal ulceration; drowsiness, headache, skin rashes and pruritus; leucopenia, urticaria and angio-oedema.

Special features
Parenteral preparations are expensive. Interaction occurs with alcohol, oral anticoagulants, phenobarbitorive and lithium.

Carbapenems

Imipenem monohydrate/cilastatin
This carbapenem/enzyme inhibitor in equal parts is useful for very severe infections or for prophylaxis. Imipenem — a thienamycin β-lactase antibiotic is administered with an enzyme inhibitor cilastatin which blocks renal inactivation for the carbapenem.

Presentation
250 mg vials
500 mg vials

Dose
250mg–1 g by intravenous infusion every 6–8 hours.
Prophylaxis: 1 g on induction of anaesthesia and 1 g 3 hours later.

Contraindications
Nil specific.

Side effects
Penicillin hypersensitivity; gastrointestinal disease, especially colitis; CNS disorders; renal dysfunction; nausea; vomiting; diarrhoea; colitis; blood dyscrasia; elevated liver enzymes, urea and creatinine; CNS disturbances; convulsions.

SUMMARY
At all times in the management of severely ill patients, the advice of the consultant microbiologist should be taken.

Naturally, the choice of antibiotic will be guided by the sensitivities of the organisms as advised by the microbiologist. Patients with a septic abortion should receive broad spectrum antibiotics against both Gram-positive and Gram-negative organisms, such as ampicillin and kanamycin, or cephaloridine and gentamicin, or carbenicillin sodium and gentamicin. The drugs should be given systemically and the uterus evacuated after 12 hours' antibiotic therapy. The dangers of septic shock should be remembered, when intravenous fluids under central venous pressure monitoring and high-dose antibiotics will be required. High-dose steroids should also be considered in the treatment of clinical septic shock.

Breast abscess

This is due to a staphylococcal infection and the antibiotic of choice is flucloxacillin sodium which is derived from the parent compound cloxacillin, but it is better absorbed. Fusidic acid (see p. 42) is an alternative preparation which may be used for penicillin-sensitive patients. Both antibiotics may be used together to prevent resistance occurring. Surgical incision and drainage of a breast abscess is rarely required.

Flucloxacillin sodium
This is a penicillin derivative.

Presentation

Capsules	250 gm, 500 mg
Syrup	125 mg/5 ml, 250 mg/5 ml
Injections	250 mg, 500 mg

Dose
An oral dose of 250 mg should be taken four times a day, or given intramuscularly or intravenously.

Contraindications
These include penicillin sensitivity.

Side effects
As for other penicillins (see p .25); it may induce cholestatic jaundice many weeks after therapy has finished.

Special features
Flucloxacillin should not be mixed with blood products or other proteinaceous fluids.

Fusidic acid, BPC
This is an alternative preparation for staphylococcal infections and those patients who are penicillin sensitive. Other antibiotics available include the cephalosporins (see p. 34) clindamycin hydrochloride (see p. 37). Fusidic acid is very active in penetrating tissue. It is excreted mainly in the bile, a minimal amount being excreted in the urine. It is not teratogenic.

Presentation

Enteric-coated tablets (each containing sodium fusidate 250 mg)	250 mg
Suspension (this preparation contains fusidic acid)	250 mg/5 ml (each 5ml is equivalent to sodium fusidate 175 mg)
Ampoules (each vial is equivalent to sodium fusidate 500 mg)	500 mg for infusion

Dose
An oral dose of 500 mg should be taken three times a day, or 500 mg given over a period of not less than 6 hours by intravenous infusion, three times daily.

Contraindications
Diethanolamine fusidate should not be given intravenously in whole blood or aminosol. It should not be given as a bolus dose or by intramuscular injection.

It should be used with caution in patients with impaired liver function.

Side effects

There are no established reports other than nausea and vomiting occurring with oral fucidate. Most adverse reactions are due to too rapid infusion of the drug.

Special features

The powder should be dissolved in the buffer provided, diluted to 250–500 ml with the infusion fluid, and infused slowly over a period of not less than 6 hours. This dosage can be given three times daily. A wide-bore vein should be chosen. The sodium content of the prepared infusion is 78.1 mmol sodium + 1.1 mmol phosphate, which is derived from the 10 ml buffer solution provided.

SUMMARY

The antibiotic of choice is the one to which the organism is sensitive. Pending sensitivities, the following may be commenced: (1) sulphafurazole or amoxycillin for urinary-tract infection; (2) co-trimoxazole, amoxycillin with clavulanic acid, tetracycline and metronidazole for pelvic inflammatory disease; (3) flucloxacillin sodium or fusidic acid for breast abscess.

Disinfection

Whereas most equipment used today may be sterilized, the most that can be done for the skin is disinfection, i.e. destruction of a large proportion of the non-sporing organisms and a small proportion of those producing spores.

Some of the agents available for skin disinfection include:

1. Soap and water — this should eliminate almost all bacteria.
2. Povidone-iodine (see p. 10) — this is compatible with soap and has the advantage over hexachlorophane of greater immediate activity.
3. Chlorhexidine — this is available as a cream for surgical scrub (chlorhexidine 3%) or for midwifery practice (chlorhexidine 1%) or as a surgical solution (chlorhexidine 4%). It has a powerful antibacterial action and is used in obstetrics as a lubricant for vaginal examinations and for application to the skin on and around the vulva and perineum during labour.
4. Ethyl alcohol 70% in water — 2 minutes' treatment will eliminate most bacteria.

5. Cetrimide, BP, Eur.P — 1% water or 0.5% in 70% alcohol — this is an alternative preparation.
6. Savlon Hospital Concentrate (ICI Pharmaceuticals) — this is a mixture of chlorhexidine gluconate solution 1.5% w/w and cetrimide 15%.

   Presentation
   25 ml sachets for direct addition to bath water as an aid to infection control.

   Dose
   Add 25 ml to 30 gallons of bath water.
7. Chloroxylenol, BP — this contains chloroxylenol 1.44% w/v and is used for pre-operative disinfection of unbroken skin.

   Presentation
   5 litre cans.

   Special features
   Chloroxylenol is also available as a concentrate of 4.8% w/w or 12% w/v mixed with ethylenediaminetetraacetic acid (EDTA). The concentrate can be made up to an aqueous alcoholic solution.
8. Benzalkonium chloride 8.0% v/v (of 50% solution); this is used in midwifery but is inactivated in the presence of soap and certain other surfactants.

Further reading

Editorial (1993). *Drug and Therapeutic Bulletin,* **31**(18). Fluoroquinolones reviewed

Mawer, G.E., Ahmad, R., Dobbs, S.M. and McGough, J.G. (1974). Prescribing for gentamicin. *British Journal of Clinical Pharmacology,* **1**, 45–50

Wise, R. (1994). *Prescribers' Journal,* **34**(3). Antibacterial agents; oral cephalosporins

Chapter 3

Infertility

Introduction

Drugs are of proven value in the management of infertile couples. Their action is either to stimulate ovulation in the female or, less successfully, to improve spermatogenesis in the male. Anti-oestrogens (including clomiphene citrate and tamoxifen citrate) may be indicated for ovulation induction if the patient is well oestrogenized and bromocriptine is used if hyperprolactinaemia is present, whilst gonadotrophin therapy is advised if there is ovarian resistance. Ovulation induction is however not without risk. The value of diet alone in returning the patient to her accepted normal weight (as defined by the life insurance company charts) should be remembered since this action alone may regulate the ovulatory menstrual cycle.

Initial investigations in any infertile couple should include a day 21 serum progesterone level, serum prolactin and serum follicle-stimulating hormone, and the patient's rubella status should be determined prior to ovulation induction. A seminal count should also be determined on one to three occasions. A basal temperature chart could be monitored to assess ovulatory function and general medical disorders should be excluded. Many patients with amenorrhoea due to anovulation may request ovulation stimulation for reassurance. Such patients should also receive adequate contraceptive advice if a pregnancy is not the primary desire. Tubal function by hysterosalpingography or laparoscopy should also be assessed.

Female infertility: induction of ovulation

1. Anti-oestrogens
    - Clomiphene citrate
    - Tamoxifen
2. Gonadotrophins
    - a) Heterologous
    - b) Homologous
        - Follicular stimulating hormone
        - Luteinising hormone

Urofollitrophin
Chorionic gonadotrophin

3. Gonadotrophin releasing hormone (GnRH) and agonists (GnRH-a)
   Gonadorelin
   Buserelin acetate
   Nafarelin
4. Dopamine agonist
   Bromocriptine
   Lysuride maleate (not available in the United States)
5. Oestrogens
6. Progestogens

Anti-oestrogens

Clomiphene citrate, BP, USP

This is a non-steroidal agent, possessing oestrogenic and anti-oestrogenic properties. It consists chemically of a mixture of *cis* and *trans* isomers of clomiphene. *cis*-Clomiphene has totally anti-oestrogenic properties in the presence of oestrogen and *trans*-clomiphene is a weak oestrogen with no anti-oestrogenic properties. *cis*-Clomiphene is available, but it has a similar ovulation rate to the racemic compound (70% of anovulatory women). It appears to act by competitively binding to the oestrogen receptor sites within the hypothalamic neurosecretory cells, thereby blocking the messenger system by which the nucleus responds to plasma oestradiol concentrations. This blockade ensures that very little oestrogen reaches the nucleus of these cells, which respond by promptly releasing gonadotrophin releasing hormone which in turn causes the release of follicle stimulating hormone from the pituitary.

Presentation

Tablets 50 mg.

Dose

Initial dose, 25–50 mg should be given daily for 5 days from day 5 of the cycle and rising to a maximum of 100 mg daily for 5 days. Other regimens begin on day 1 or day 3 of the cycle.

Contraindications

Clomiphene citrate is not recommended by the manufacturers during pregnancy, and hence a second course should not be continued should a pregnancy test prove positive. There is, however, no evidence that clomiphene citrate has a harmful effect on the human fetus, but it does damage rat and rabbit fetuses in high dosage. Liver disease or a history of liver dysfunction is also a contraindication, as is abnormal uterine bleeding.

Indications
Clomiphene citrate is recommended to stimulate ovulation in the polycystic ovary syndrome and also for patients suffering from 'post-Pill amenorrhoea'. It has also been used for men with a low sperm count.

Side effects
Those reported include hot flushes, loss of hair, Mittelschmerz (mid-cycle ovulation pain), blurring of vision, lower abdominal pain, ovarian enlargement and multiple pregnancy (incidence 8%). Ovarian malignancy has been reported after prolonged use (Rossing M.A. et al.).

Special features
No 25 mg tablet is manufactured, but the 50 mg tablets are scored. Many clinicians use as much as 200 mg daily although a maximum of 150 mg is now recommended. No hormone studies are required before the initiation of therapy. The 25 mg dose should be used if there is evidence of polycystic ovarian disease, and human chorionic gonadotrophin may be used with clomiphene citrate to improve the luteal phase. Day 21 progesterone estimations or ultrasound are performed to confirm ovulation. Failure to conceive after 6 months' therapy suggests the need for gonadotrophin therapy. There have been recent reports of an increase in the incidence of neural tube defects in the offspring; also the potential for ovarian malignancy following high dose regimes of over 12 months has been reported.

Tamoxifen citrate
This may be effective in patients who do not respond to clomiphene citrate. The preparation is related to clomiphene citrate but, in contrast, the *trans* isomer has ovulation-inducing properties. In high doses it has direct oestrogenic activity. Any abnormal bleeding *per uteri* needs evaluating as cases of endometrial cancer have been reported in patients on tamoxifen.

Like clomiphene citrate (see p. 46) it competes with oestrogen for specific receptor sites in the genital tract and anterior pituitary.

Presentation
Tablets 10 mg, 20 mg, 40 mg.

Dose
An oral dose of 20 mg should be taken daily on days 2–5 of the menstrual cycle, rising to 40 mg and a maximum of 80 mg twice daily.

Contraindications
These include pregnancy.

Indications
It is recommended for patients suffering from anovulatory infertility.

Side effects
Those reported include ovarian swelling, hot flushes, vaginal bleeding, pruritus vulvae, gastrointestinal intolerance, lightheadedness, fluid retention and transient falls in platelet count.

Special features
Interaction with warfarin occurs.

Gonadotrophins (heterologous and homologous)

The biggest disadvantage of *heterologous gonadotrophins* is the ability to produce antihormones with cross-reaction to human gonadotrophin. They are of no use for inducing ovulation in humans.

The *homologous gonadotrophins* include a mixture of follicle-stimulating hormone (FSH) and luteinising hormone (LH), with a predominantly FSH action. Inter-batch variation in biological activity may occur and research continues to produce highly pure FSH preparations (see p. 49). These are in short supply and, in the UK, human menopausal gonadotrophin produced from menopausal urine is more readily available. They control the growth and maturation of the ovarian follicle and together with human chorionic gonadotrophin hCG are used in hypopituitarism; they are also used in assisted reproductive programmes.

Human menopausal gonadotrophins, (metrodin and metrodin-HP)
Both the above drugs are obtained from urine of menopausal women and the starting source of both the drugs is human menopausal gonadotrophin (hmg).

Hmg injections ('Humegon' Organon) are a mixture of both the natural gonadotrophins, hFSH (human follicle stimulating hormone) and LH (luteinising hormone) with activity available in strengths of 75 IU or 150 IU respectively per ampoule ('Pergonal' Serono is available only in 75 IU ampoules). The hLH activity is provided by appropriate amounts of hCG hormone, (generally 3.7 mg–10.2 mg of hCG providing 75 IU of hLH activity). 95% of the proteins in such preparations are inactive urinary proteins.

The pure FSH preparations available have an improved FSH activity of 100–200 IU of FSH activity per mg protein. However, the highly purified compound (Metrodin HP) contains FSH activity of up to 9000 IU/mg protein. This is achieved by using immunoaffinity chromatography with an anti-FSH monoclonal antibody. Further purification steps include reversed-phase high pressure liquid chromatography and QAE-sepharose chromatography.

Advantages of high-purity FSH

1. Metrodin HP can be administered as a subcutaneous injection with no difference in pharmacokinetics as compared to the intramuscular route.
2. The high concentrations of LH during the late follicular phase are postulated to cause a decrease in fertilization rates and an increase in the miscarriage rates in women with polycystic ovarian syndrome (PCOS). Pure FSH is postulated to allow a better stimulation and thus success in the management of polycystic ovaries. Some studies, however, have shown no significant advantage of high purity FSH (Metrodin HP) over HMG in increasing pregnancy rates or reducing hyperstimulation syndromes or multiple births.

Dose

Schedule 1: daily intramuscular injections of 75 units are given for 3 days, rising to 150 units for up to 7 days until a satisfactory oestrogenic response is seen; the injections are followed by a single injection of human chorionic gonadotrophin (hCG), 10,000 units 2 days after the last dose of menotrophin (Pergonal).

Schedule 2: three injections of equal amounts of menotrophin (Pergonal) (150–225 units) are given on alternate days (days 1, 3, 5), followed by hCG, 10,000 units, on day 8 to trigger ovulation and corpus luteum formation.

The Pergonal will simply stimulate follicular development and the hCG is given to provide an ovulatory surge of LH.

Contraindications

The following should be excluded or treated before commencing treatment: ovarian dysgenesis and premature menopause; myxoedema or adrenal abnormality; pituitary tumour; ovarian tumour.

Side effects

These include pyrexia, pains in the joints, local injection-site reactions, ovarian hyperstimulation and multiple pregnancy (the incidence can be reduced by strict monitoring of follicular development with ultrasound and oestrogen values). The full-blown ovarian hyperstimulation syndrome can lead to death. There is a shift of albumin from the plasma to the peritoneal cavity resulting in ascites, hypokalaemia, haemoconcentration, circulatory failure and thrombosis which is often arterial. Treatment should be prompt with intravenous fluid, albumin and abdominal paracentesis. Laparotomy should be strictly avoided unless there is evidence of bleeding. The ovaries may enlarge to above the umbilicus, but will regress within 28 days. The syndrome is extremely rare and it is not essential to assess the ovarian size after each monthly cycle.

Special features

Professional laboratory services will undertake oestrogen assays and report the results within 24 hours of receipt of the specimens if local assay facilities are not available. Ultrasound monitoring of follicular size is mandatory — hCG should not be given if three follicles are present larger than 16 mm.The gonadotrophin dose is altered on the basis of ovarian response to avoid multiple pregnancy.

Side effects

The major side effect is the hyperstimulation syndrome (ovarian enlargement; low abdominal pain; ascites) (see p. 49).

Urofollitrophin (FSH)

This is almost pure follicle-stimulating hormone.

Presentation

Freeze-dried powder in ampoules 75 IU.

Dose

75–150 IU daily, or 225–375 IU on alternate days by i.m. injection.
Dose to be adjusted until desired response monitored by oestrogen levels or ultrasonography achieved.

Contraindications

Pregnancy.

Side effects

Sensitivity reactions; ovarian hyperstimulation, enlargement and rupture; multiple pregnancy.

Special features

Intracranial disorder and endocrine disorders should be treated pre-therapy.

Chorionic gonadotrophin, BP, USP (human chorionic gonadotrophin, hCG)

The biological properties of human chorionic gonadotrophins are very similar to those of luteinising hormone. Human chorionic gonadotrophins are capable of inducing ovulation after a follicle has been developed, converting it to corpus luteum. HCG is extracted from pregnant women's urine and is more readily available than luteinising hormone.

Presentation

Injection	500 units/ml
	1,000 units/ml
	1,500 units/ml

2,000 units/ml
5,000 units/ml
10,000 units/ml

Dose
An intramuscular injection of 3,000–10,000 units of hCG should be given at a time dependent on the oestrogen response value after human menopausal gonadotrophin therapy or clomiphene citrate therapy.

Contraindications
Oestrogen values should be monitored after human menopausal gonadotrophin therapy and hCG only given if the patient is not over-responding. This will reduce the possibilities of multiple pregnancy. HCG should not be given if absolute values of 140 μg/24 hours total oestrogen, 60 μg/24 hours total oestrone or 70 μg/24 hours total oestriol are exceeded. (Alternative units may be used in individual laboratories.) To avoid multiple pregnancy, hCG should not be given if there are more than three ovarian follicles larger than 16 mm on ultrasound scan or if follicular maturation is excessive (see above).

Indications
HCG is advised for the management of patients with anovulation and is given in association with human menopausal gonadotrophin. It may be given as luteal support.

Gonadotrophin releasing hormones (GnRH) and analogues (GnRH-a) (see p. 66)

Gonadorelin (GHRH)
This is a gonadotrophin-releasing hormone analogue.

Presentation
Injection of 500 μg/ml.

Dose
Determined individually.

Contraindications
Endometriosis; polycystic ovary disease; weight-related amenorrhoea before correction of weight loss.

Side effects
Abdominal pain, nausea, headache, menorrhagia.

Special features
Discontinue after conception or before 6 months.

Buserelin acetate

This is a gonadotrophin-releasing hormone analogue. It is used prior to *in vitro* fertilization protocols to down regulate the pituitary gland and prevent premature surge of LH (luteinising hormone).

Presentation

Nasal spray 150 μg per dose.

Dose

Determined individually.

Contraindications

Pregnancy; lactation; undiagnosed vaginal bleeding; hormone-dependent neoplasm.

Side effects

Hot flushes; vaginal dryness; loss of libido; emotional lability; headache; breast tenderness; local nasal irritation.

Special features

It interacts with nasal decongestants and prolonged use may lead to osteoporosis.

Ovulation induction for *in vivo* fertilization and embryo transfer

Gonadotrophin releasing hormones (GnRH) analogues in In vitro fertilization (IVF) [buserelin (Suprecur), nafarelin (Synarel)]

Mechanism of action

These act by down regulation of the pituitary receptors for GnRH. The initial action is of stimulation of the pituitary, which causes release of the pituitary gonadotrophins. Subsequently, however, there is desensitization of the pituitary due to their prolonged stimulation and thus the FSH and LH concentrations decrease. This prevents follicles from developing and thus creates a hypo-oestrogenic state. The ovaries, however, are responsive to external gonadotrophins. Thus, in IVF cycles, the use of GnRH-analogues can allow better control of the follicle stimulation without the fear of spontaneous LH surge from the pituitary. This also avoids the need for repeated assays for LH surge which used to be such a prominent feature of IVF cycles in the past.

Chemistry

In the decapeptide structure of GnRH, one or more amino acids are substituted with synthetic acids which are relatively resistant to breakdown by peptidase enzymes.

Presentation and dose

Suprecur (buserelin acetate) is available in bottles of 2 x 100 metred dose-units; each dose is of 150 μg. It must be sniffed every 6 hours and the last nightly dose is two sniffs to be taken just before bedtime.

Synarel (nafarelin) is a longer acting compound and is to be sniffed twice daily (200 μg per dose, 60 metred dose-units).

Indications

In assisted conception cycles needing superovulation (IVF *et al.*). Polycystic ovarian syndrome resistant to induction of ovulation by clomiphene citrate can be treated using low-dose gonadotrophin regimes, and some clinicians use GnRH-analogues in addition, with these regimes.

Contraindications

Pregnancy and lactation are the obvious contraindications. Known nasal allergy to the compound is another.

The 'long protocol' and the 'short protocol' ('flare-up protocol') of GnRH-analogues in IVF

As mentioned earlier, the chief advantage of using GnRH-analogues in superovulation regimes for IVF is that they give a more predictable, controlled ovarian stimulation, and oocyte retrieval can be better planned as spontaneous LH surge is reliably avoided. There have been some studies showing that regimes using GnRH-analogues (as compared to those using gonadotrophins alone) have more oocytes recovered, but this is not the main reason for the inclusion of this drug in stimulation regimes.

The 'long protocol' starts from the 21st day of the previous cycle. The inhalation of GnRH-analogues down regulates the pituitary and the ovaries become quiescent; this normally takes between 2 and 3 weeks of treatment. Commonly, the patient has a menstrual period a few days after commencing sniffing of the GnRH-analogue. Ovarian suppression can be confirmed by doing a baseline trans-vaginal scan or from serum oestradiol levels below 50–100 picomoles/l (each centre and laboratory have their own variations). Gonadotrophin injections are then commenced while inhalation of the GnRH-analogue continues to prevent a spontaneous ovarian surge later in the cycle. The GnRH-analogue is stopped only after giving the trigger injection of hCG.

The 'short protocol' ('flare-up protocol')

This protocol involves sniffing of the GnRH-analogue for a much shorter duration. It takes advantage of the initial burst of gonadotrophins that immediately follows the start of GnRH-analogue treatment. On the second day of a menstrual period, there is a physiological elevation of FSH as the follicles for the new cycle are recruited. GnRH-analogue treatment is commenced at this point (day 1 or 2), so that the 'flare up' of gonadotrophins augments the physiological elevation of FSH and a greater number of follicles are recruited. Human menopausal gonadotrophins are commenced soon after (day 3) so that there are sustained elevated FSH levels. The later parts of the management of the cycle are similar to the 'long protocol' described above. The short protocol shortens the period of treatment and the number of ampoules of gonadotrophins and thus reduces costs.

Clinical success for both the above protocols is similar. The advantage of the long protocol is that it gives better control over follicular stimulation.

Side effects
Headaches are often seen following GnRH-analogue sniffing. Local reaction with allergy-like symptoms and a feeling of bloatedness can occur. Hot flushes are common. Ovarian cysts are often seen following this treatment. Some reports have revealed more incidence of ovarian hyperstimulation syndrome following this treatment. Bone loss with GnRH-analogues is not relevant when a compound is used with superovulation regimes. The occurrence of a pregnancy when sniffing GnRH-analogues is seen in the occasional patient planned for IVF treatment. Though tubal pregnancies have been reported in some such cases, there is no evidence that the GnRG-analogue has a causal role. There have been no obvious teratogenic effects on babies in such pregnancies. There is an adverse luteolytic effect of continued GnRH-a administration on the progression of early pregnancy.

Dopamine agonists

Bromocriptine mesylate (see p. 158)

This is indicated for the management of female infertility in patients who normally suffer from amenorrhoea including lactational amenorrhoea, and galactorrhoea, and who have an elevated serum prolactin value. It is a dopamine agonist and controls prolactin secretion mainly at pituitary level. A pituitary fossa radiograph to exclude an enlarging pituitary tumour is indicated if hyperprolactinaemia is found. Normal values of prolactin vary in different laboratories and local values need to be determined (normally in excess of 400 μg). The assay may vary throughout the 24-hour time span and bromocriptine may be given empirically with normal prolactin levels. Hyperprolactincemia can be associated with hypothyroidism and thyroid function should be evaluated.

Presentation

Tablets	1.0 mg, 2.5 mg
Capsules	5 mg, 10 mg

Dose

An oral dose of 1.25 mg at night, increasing the dose gradually to reduce the initial side effects (see below). Maximum dose 30 mg daily.

Contraindications

No absolute contraindications are known. Hypersensitivity to ergot alkaloids. Use with caution with history of psychotic or severe cardiovascular disorders.

Indications

Hyperprolactinaemic anovulation. Bromocriptine is also of value for the suppression of lactation (see p. 158) and for the management of galactorrhoea.

Side effects

Nausea, postural hypotension, dizziness, headache, vomiting and mild constipation have been reported; retroperitoneal fibrosis, dry mouth or leg cramps. Digital vasospasm. Rarely hypertension. Myocardial infarction, cerebrovascular accidents, drowsiness, confusion, hallucinations, headache, dizziness, seizures.

Special features

If hyperprolactinaemia is diagnosed, the visual fields should be assessed and a pituitary fossa radiograph obtained. Should a pituitary fossa tumour be diagnosed, referral to a specialist centre is mandatory. Many drugs affect the release of prolactin and thus affect the assay (Table 3.1) It interacts with alcohol, erythromycin, metoclopramide and hypotensives.

Lysuride maleate

This is a dopaminergic agent which lowers physiologically and pathologically elevated prolactin levels and growth hormone levels. It is said to be the most potent prolactin-lowering agent so far known and is mainly available in Europe. It is marketed in the UK for parkinsonism.

Oestrogens (estrogens)

Prior to clomiphene citrate and gonadotrophin therapy, oestrogens were used for the induction of ovulation. However, oestrogens are now only advised to antagonize the anti-oestrogen effect of clomiphene citrate, especially in patients showing evidence of poor cervical mucus and sperm penetration on a post-coital test.

Presentation

Tablets ethinyloestradiol 10 μg
equine oestrogens — conjugated (Premarin; Wyeth) 0.625 mg
oestriol 0.25 mg

Table 3.1 Substances influencing prolactin release

Substances with prolactin-inhibiting properties

L-dopa
Dopamine agonists
- bromocriptine
- lergotrile
- lysuride (not available in the United States)
- methergoline
- apomorphine
- piribedil

Substances which stimulate secretion of prolactin

Neuroleptics
- phenothiazines
- butyrophenones
- thioxanthenes

Antidepressants
- dibenzazepine derivatives (in high doses)
- imipramine

Antihypertensives
- α-methyldopa
- reserpine

Hormones and antagonists
- oestrogens
- oral contraceptives
- protirelin

Opiates
- morphine
- methadone

Antihistamines
- meclozine

H_2-receptor blockers
- cimetidine

Anti-emetics
- metoclopramide
- thiethylperazine (not available in the United States)

Others
- baclofen (not available in the United States)

Dose
Ethinyloestradiol 10 µg should be given from days 9 to 12 or Premarin 0.625 mg from days 9 to 12; oestriol 0.25–1 mg is given daily on days 6 to15 of the cycle.

Contraindications
They should be used with caution in patients suffering from epilepsy, migraine, asthma or cardiac and renal disease owing to salt and water retention. They should not be given to patients with a history of thromboembolism/ thrombophlebitis or breast and genital cancers.

Indications
They are advised to improve the cervical mucus in patients taking clomiphene citrate but having a negative post-coital test.

Side effects
These include salt and water retention, and thrombotic problems. If given too early in the cycle, oestrogens may inhibit ovulation.

Special features
None.

Progestogens

These have been used to supplement the luteal phase from day 15 of ovulation.

Presentation
Vaginal pessary Cyclogest 200 mg; 400 mg
Injection 25mg Gestone
Tablets

Dydrogesterol	10 mg
Medroxyprogesterone	5 mg; 10 mg

Side effects
Gastrointestinal upset; skin and mucous membrane reactions; breast tenderness; galactorrhoea; weight gain.

SUMMARY

To stimulate ovulation, anti-oestrogens are advised and initially clomiphene citrate is recommended. If the serum prolactin level is elevated, then bromocriptine should be prescribed. Failure to stimulate ovulation with these agents will necessitate the use of gonadotrophins or gonadotrophin releasing hormone.

Male infertility: improvement of spermatogenesis

In 30% of infertile couples the male partner is at fault, due to azoospermia or oligospermia. The normal semen analysis has a semen count of more than 20 million sperms per ml, a normal motility at 6 hours of 40% progressive activity and at least 40% of sperms with normal morphology (see Table 3.2).

The management of oligoasthenic semen is unsatisfactory, as illustrated by the various medications available, but until further research elucidates the aetiology(ies) of oligospermia, spermatokinetic agents may be tried; however, they should be given for a minimum of 100 days, since maturation of spermatogenesis takes 80 days. They should be given for no longer than 12 months. Their value is restricted and the management of oligospermia includes empirical advice (loose underwear, low scrotal temperature), antibiotics, ligature of varicocoele, correction of endocrine abnormalities and concentration of fresh semen and subsequent artificial insemination or even artificial insemination using donor semen. Advances in andrology now allow intracytoplasmic sperm injection.

Variable successes have been reported with arginine hydrochloride, clomiphene citrate, fluoxymesterone, and mesterolone, which has been advocated for patients with semen showing low motility. In the present state of knowledge it should be remembered that placebos may be as successful as alternative therapy.

Mesterolone

This is an orally active androgen which does not cause pituitary suppression at the recommended dosage and endogenous androgen production is unaffected. It is thought to stimulate spermatogenesis by supplementing deficient testicular androgens, thus improving both sperm count and motility.

Presentation

Tablets 25 mg.

Table 3.2 Semen analysis — Normal values (WHO)

Volume	2–5 ml
Liquefaction time	within 30 minutes
Concentration	20–200 million spermatozoa per ml
Motility	greater than 40% motile (grades I and II)
Morphology	greater than 40% normal forms

Dose
An oral dose of 25 mg should be taken four times a day for a maximum of 12 months.

Contraindications
These include prostatic carcinoma or hepatic carcinoma.

Side effects
Those reported have included hepatic carcinoma and priapism.

Special features
None.

Further reading

Anyso, N. (1993) *The Control and Stimulation of Follicular Growth* (ed. R. Shaw) Chapter 14, Parthenon Publishing Group.

Casper, R.F. and Yen, S.S.C. (1979) Induction of luteolysis in the human with a long acting analog of luteinising hormone releasing factor. *Science*, **205**, pp.408–410.

Cuckle, H., Walo, N. (1989) Ovulation induction and neural tube defects. *Lancet,* pp.2–128.

Czeizel, A. (1989) Ovulation induction and neural tube defects. *Lancet,* pp. 2–167

Howles, C. (1990). Gonadotrophin releasing hormone analogues; past, present and future uses in superovulation regime, in *Clinical IVF Forum.* (ed. P.L. Matson and B.A. Lieberman). Manchester University Press, Manchester, pp. 41–42.

Hull, M.G.R. (1991). G*onadotrophins, Gonadotrophin Releasing Hormone Analogues and Growth Factors in Infertility. Future Perspectives* (ed. C.M. Howles). pp. 56–69.

Royal College of Obstetricians and Gynaecologists, London. *Guidelines: Use of gonadotrophic hormone preparations for ovulation induction,* No. 2, April 1994.

Rossing A.A. et al. (1994) Ovarian tumors in a cohort of infertile women. *New England Journal of Medicine* (1994), **331**, pp. 771–776.

Shane, J.M. (1993) Evaluation and Treatment of Infertility Clinical Symposia Vol 45 No.2 Ciba.

Chapter 4

Dysmenorrhoea and Endometriosis

Introduction

It is still useful to distinguish two types of period pain as primary, congestive or ovulatory dysmenorrhoea and dysmenorrhoea secondary to pelvic inflammatory disease or endometriosis. There may be considerable overlap between the two varieties.

Primary dysmenorrhoea

Primary, spasmodic, congestive dysmenorrhoea is associated with ovulation, and menstrual fluid from ovulatory cycles has high levels of prostaglandins. The severe pain can be associated with gastrointestinal upsets, nausea, vomiting, diarrhoea and headache, necessitating loss of time from work or study. Uterine abnormalities such as bicornuate uterus or early pregnancy should be considered, otherwise treatment can be empirical with mild analgesics and psychotherapy and supportive measures including anti-emetics or mild heat. More specific treatments include ovulation suppression with a low-dose oral contraceptive, but other alternatives include progestogens or antiprostaglandins including aspirin, indomethacin or mefenamic acid.

Oestrogen–progestogen combinations (see p. 145)

A low-dose combined oestrogen–progestogen preparation should be prescribed.

Presentation
Combination tablets, e.g. ethinyloestradiol 0.03 mg, levonorgestrel 0.15 mg.

Dose
One tablet daily for 21 days starting on day 5.

Contraindications
See p. 146.

Side effects
See p. 149.

Special features
A full description of oestrogen–progestogen combinations is given in Appendix I; many young patients may present with dysmenorrhoea, although indirectly their primary request may be for oral contraception.

Progestogens

Dydrogesterone, BP
This progestogen has been shown to relieve dysmenorrhoea without inhibiting ovulation and can be used for patients with oligomenorrhoea.

Presentation
Tablets 10 mg.

Dose
One tablet should be taken three times a day, from days 5 to 25 of each menstrual cycle, for a minimum of three-to-four cycles.

Contraindications
None known.

Side effects
Breakthrough bleeding can occur, which can be controlled by increasing the dose.

Special features
There is no virilization of the fetus should the patient become pregnant. The drug is also used in the medical treatment of endometriosis (see p. 65).

Norethisterone BP (norethindrone, USP) (see p. 64)

Presentation
Tablets 5 mg.

Dose
One tablet should be taken three times a day for 20 days, starting on day 5 of each cycle, for three-to-four cycles.

Non-steroidal anti-inflammatory drugs (see Table 5.1, Chapter 5)

Many non-steroidal anti-inflammatory drugs are antiprostaglandins (see p. 69) and they include, amongst others, aspirin, indomethacin and mefenamic acid.

Aspirin BP, Eur.P, USP (acetylsalicylic acid)

There are many preparations available, either solo or in combination packs, which are to be discouraged. Aspirin is best dispensed as soluble aspirin (soluble aspirin, BP) to reduce gastric irritation.

Presentation

Tablets 300 mg.

Dose

An oral dose of one-to-three tablets every 4 hours (max 12 tabs/day).

Contraindications

Active peptic ulceration or allergy to aspirin.

Side effects

Aspirin may precipitate bronchospasm and asthma in susceptible subjects; it may induce gastrointestinal haemorrhage and enhance the effect of anticoagulants.

Special features

Aspirin interacts with other drugs and a specific hazard is warfarin interaction (see Table 10.3 Chapter 10).

Indomethacin, BP

Presentation

Capsules	25 mg, 50 mg, 75 mg, sustained release
Suspension	25 mg/5 ml
Suppositories	100 mg

Dose

An oral dose of 25 mg every 6 hours for 48–72 hours, or 100 mg suppository every 6 hours for 49–72 hours, or 75 mg sustained release, once or twice daily (max daily dose indomethacin = 200 mg ie, 100 mg bd prn).

Contraindications

Active peptic ulcer, gastrointestinal lesions and sensitivity to indomethacin.

Side effects

Nausea, vomiting and dyspepsia. Maculopapular eruptions may occur.

Special features

The suppositories may be of value if the patient is vomiting or nauseous, but tenesmus, proctitis, rectal bleeding, pain, discomfort and itching have all been reported following their use.

Mefenamic acid, BP

This is an analgesic with anti-inflammatory, antipyretic and anti-prostaglandin activity.

Presentation

Tablets	500 mg
Capsules	250 mg
Suspension	50 mg/5 ml

Dose

An oral dose of 500 mg three times a day.

Contraindications

Patients with inflammatory bowel disease or suffering from peptic and/or intestinal ulceration, and patients with renal or hepatic impairment.

Side effects

May affect the dosage of concurrent anticoagulant therapy. Diarrhoea may occur within 24 hours of starting therapy; skin rashes; allergic glomerulonephritis and rarely thrombocytopenia have all been reported. Reversible haemolytic anaemia and temporary lowering of white blood cell count have been reported and bronchospasm may be precipitated in patients suffering from, or with a previous history of, bronchial asthma or allergic disease. Rarely, drowsiness and dizziness have been reported.

Special features

Mefenamic acid is also of value for patients with dysfunctional uterine haemorrhage (see p. 69).

Antispasmodics

Hyoscine-N-butyl bromide

This is an antispasmodic agent which relaxes smooth muscle and is believed to act on the intramural parasympathetic ganglia of the organs.

Presentation

Tablets	10 mg
Injections	20 mg/ml

Dose

An oral dose of two tablets three times a day, commencing 2 days prior to the expected date of the menstrual period and continuing for 5 days.

Contraindications

Patients with glaucoma.

Side effects
Dry mouth, temporary loss of accommodation and tachycardia.

Special features
The drug is also used in the management of the premenstrual syndrome (see p. 77).

Summary
The incidence of primary dysmenorrhoea has declined considerably during the past 20 years; it is associated with ovulation, and oral contraceptives should act as a cure. Occasionally, this therapy is declined by the patient (or parent) and alternative drug regimes, including antiprostaglandin therapy, should be tried. Rarely, dilatation of the cervix with possible laparoscopy to exclude other pathology will be required.

Secondary dysmenorrhoea

Dysmenorrhoea secondary to local causes such as pelvic inflammation, endometriosis, fibroids or the presence of an intra-uterine device, is initially treated by establishing the diagnosis, normally by laparoscopy, and then applying appropriate therapy. Where dysmenorrhoea is secondary to endometriosis, therapy may be combined surgical and medical therapy or medical therapy alone, which will involve progestogens, combined oestrogen–progestogen preparations, danazol therapy or gonadotrophin-releasing hormone analogues.

Progestogens

These are used to create a state of pseudo-pregnancy and they improve endometriosis both clinically and histologically by inducing a decidual reaction in the endometrium.

Norethisterone, BP (norethindrone, USP)
This is used in the management of dysfunctional uterine haemorrhage (see p. 72), premenstrual syndrome (see p. 76), dysmenorrhoea and endometriosis.

Presentation
Tablets 5 mg

Dose
A daily dose of 10 mg from day 5 of each cycle; the dose may be increased to 25 mg daily if intermenstrual bleeding occurs. For endometriosis it should be given continuously.

Contraindications
Pregnancy (which in itself is a cure for endometriosis); severe disturbance of liver function; Dubin–Johnson and Rotor syndromes; previous history during pregnancy of idiopathic jaundice, severe pruritus or herpes gestation.

Side effects
Nausea, exacerbation of epilepsy and migraine; cholestatic liver changes in high dosage.

Special features
The drug is relatively cheap.

Dydrogesterone, BP (see p. 61)

Medroxyprogesterone acetate
This preparation is used as a contraceptive (see p. 152); in malignancy (see p. 164); and for dysfunctional menstruation and endometriosis. It allows a prompt return to ovulation after treatment.

Presentation

Tablets	5 mg, 10 mg
Injection	50 mg/ml

Dose
For endometriosis, 10 mg t.d.s. for 90 days beginning on first day of the menstrual cycle.

Contraindications
Thromboembolic disease; liver dysfunction; genital or breast neoplasm.

Side effects
Progestogenic effects (see above).

Special features
Care should be used in patients with epilepsy, migraine, asthma, cardiac or renal dysfunction, diabetes or depression. Exclude genital malignancy and pregnancy before use.

Combined oestrogen–progestogen preparations (see p. 145)

This treatment is still widely used, especially with pelvic inflammation.

Danazol

This synthetic steroid is derived from ethisterone and controls pituitary gonadotrophin output without any concomitant oestrogenic or progestational activity of its own. The true mode of action of danazol has still to be elucidated.

Presentation
Capsules 100 mg, 200 mg.

Dose
A daily dose of 200–800 mg should be taken daily for up to 6 months.

Contraindications
Nil specific (except pregnancy).

Side effects
Fluid retention, flushing, skin rashes, hirsutism and rarely clitoral hypertrophy. Danazol may increase insulin resistance and aggravate diabetes mellitus. It may potentiate anticoagulants and care is required in patients with hepatic dysfunction. Other adverse reactions reported include: nervousness and nauseous headache, dizziness, vertigo, emotional lability, backache, skeletal muscle spasm, hair loss, weight gain and voice changes.

Special features
Danazol can inhibit ovulation, but should not be relied on for contraception. Non-hormonal methods for contraception should be used, since oestrogen–progestogens can modify the action of danazol. Danazol in low dosage (100 mg on alternate days throughout the cycle) is also of value in the management of premenstrual syndrome (see p. 76) or menorrhagia (see p. 77). Danazol is also advocated to render the endometrium atrophic prior to endometrial resection: 200 mg of danazol is given t.d.s. for 6 weeks prior to surgery.

Gonadotrophin releasing hormone (GnRH) and agonists (see p. 51)

Introduction
GnRH is a decapeptide produced by the arcuate nucleus of the hypothalamus. The hormone is secreted in pulses and controls the release of both FSH and LH from the pituitary. In recent years, 'GnRH pumps' have come into vogue for the treatment of amenorrhoea of hypothalamic etiology. However, this treatment is quite cumbersome and the indications are limited.

The molecule of GnRH assumes a hairpin structure making the amino acids 6 and 7 most vulnerable for degradation by pituitary endopeptidases. The amino acids 9 and 10 are cleaved by a carboxyamide peptidase and the action of the above enzymes is responsible for the very short half life of GnRH (of 2–8 minutes). The development of GnRH analogues however makes good clinical use of the knowledge of the structure of GnRH itself. These compounds are resistant to the peptidases and thus have a prolonged half-life. They cause a reversible suppression of the pituitary following an initial burst of LH and FSH secretion. These new drugs have found extensive use in gynaecology as well as in the management of prostatic and breast cancer as in effect they cause 'medical castration'. The GnRH-analogues available for inhalation are the shorter acting compounds [Buserelin 'Suprecur' (Hoechst). Nafarelin 'Synarel (Syntex)] generally used in super-ovulation regimes (IVF etc.), while the injectables are depot preparations [Goserelin acetate, 'Zoladex', Zeneca), (Leuprorelin acetate, 'Prostap SR', Lederle)] lasting for approximately one month, are generally used in other indications such as treatment of endometriosis and cancers (breast and prostate). This classification of routes and uses is however not rigid.

The mechanism of action of the drug by either routes is the same.

Presentation

Buserelin nasal spray (not available in the United States)
Nafarelin nasal spray
Goserelin depot preparation for subcutaneous injection
Leuprorelin depot preparation for subcutaneous injection

Dose

Buserelin	900 μg/die (two 150 μg sprays t.d.s.)
Nafarelin	400 μg/die (one 200 μg spray b.d.)
Goserelin	3.6 mg base by s.c. injection into abdominal wall every 28 days. Max duration of treatment 6 months
Leuprorelin	3.75 mg as s.c. injection or intramuscular injections every 28 days. Max duration of treatment 6 months

Contraindications

Pregnancy or lactating woman, or vaginal bleeding of unknown origin.

Side effects

Menopausal symptoms (see p. 80). Loss of bone density after 6 months' use.

Special features

Best reserved for patients who cannot tolerate unwanted effects of other treatments; if used, restrict to single 6 months' course. They have also been used as adjunctive therapy prior to myomectomy, hysterectomy, or endometrial resection or ablation.

Further reading

Bromham, D.R. (1993). Update in endometriosis. *Postgraduate Update*, 1 March 1993.

Goldrath, M.H. (1990). *Journal of Reproductive Medicine*, **35**(1) (Supplement), 91–96.

Hawkins, D.F. (1992). Symposium on Medical Treatment of Chronic Pelvic Pain. *Journal of Obstetrics and Gynaecology*, **12** (Supplement 2), November 1992.

Herzl M.R. (1988). *Clinical Obstetrics and Gynaecology* **31**(4); Gonadotrophin releasing hormone (GnRH) agonist in the management of endometriosis; a review.

Leading Article. Gonadotrophin releasing hormone analogue for endometriosis. *Drug and Therapeutics Bulletin*, **31**(6), Consumers' Association, 15 March 1993.

Metzger, D.A. and Luciano A.A. (1989). *Obstetrics and Gynaecology Clinics of North America*, **16**(1). 105–122.

Schweppe K.W. (1990) Current medical therapies for endometriosis — a review. *Endometriosis* Volume 1. *Advances in Reproductive Endocrinology*. Parthenon, UK, p. 67.

Zuspan, F .P. and Christian, C.D. (1983). *Controversy in Obstetrics and Gynaecology*, Volume III, ch. 20. W.B. Saunders, London, pp. 7–47.

Chapter 5

Dysfunctional Uterine Haemorrhage

Introduction

Numerous ill-defined terms have been used to describe varieties of dysfunctional uterine haemorrhage, such as menorrhagia (hypermenorrhoea), epimenorrhagia (polymenorrhagia) and metrostaxis (metrorrhagia). In reality, periods may be too long, too frequent, too profuse or too irregular.

Dysfunctional uterine haemorrhage implies a hormonal imbalance causing an irregular menstrual cycle. It is a clinical diagnosis that may be made when general and pelvic examinations (including hysteroscopy and laparoscopy) reveal no abnormality to account for recurrent and excessive bleeding per vaginum. Studies suggest 80–90% of patients with regular periods have no hormone imbalance. *Organic pathology must be excluded.*

Non-hormonal preparations can be used to regulate the menstrual loss, and associated iron deficiency anaemia will require appropriate haematinic therapy.

Treatment

Non-steroidal anti-inflammatory drugs (NSAIDs) (see Table 5.1)

Based on studies demonstrating an excess of prostaglandins in the endometrium from patients with dysfunctional uterine bleeding, NSAIDS (antiprostaglandins) including mefenamic acid (see p. 63) or flufenamic acid have been tried with reasonable success. The prostaglandins in the endometrium are thought to cause an increased blood flow through vasodilatation of the spiral arterioles in the myometrium and basal layer of the endometrium. There is also inhibition of platelet aggregation. The uterine contractions associated with primary dysmenorrhoea and produced by prostaglandins are also inhibited.

Table 5.1 Non-Steroidal anti-inflammatory drugs (NSAIDs)

Aspirin and salicylates

Ibuprofen and propionic acid derivatives

Miscellaneous drugs with properties similar to those of propionic acid derivatives

azapropazone
diclofenac
diflunisal
etodolac
indomethacin
mefenamic acid (see p. 63)
nabumetone
phenylbutazone
sulindac
tolmetin

The main differences between NSAIDs are in the incidence and type of side effects; there is considerable individual patient response and several drugs may be tried before finding one to suit a particular patient; mefenamic acid is specifically marketed for dysmenorrhoea and dysfunctional bleeding.

Systemic haemostats

Ethamsylate

This is a systemic haemostat. The mode of action of ethamsylate is unknown, but it is thought to have a specific tissue receptor in the vessel and capillary walls and having once located this receptor it exerts a protective action against breakdown by histamine, hyaluronidase and possibly the kinin system. It may also inhibit the biosynthesis and action of the prostaglandins which cause platelet disaggregation, vasodilation and increased capillary permeability.

Presentation

Injections	250 mg/2 ml
Tablets	500 mg

Dose

An oral dose of 500 mg should be taken four times a day; it should be started from the time bleeding starts until menstruation ceases; the use before the bleeding starts is not recommended.

Contraindications
None known.

Side effects
Occasional headaches or skin rashes.

Special features
The drug has no effect on the endometrial histology should curettage subsequently be required. Ethamsylate is also advocated for the prevention and treatment of periventricular haemorrhage in low birth weight infants. It is not available in the United States.

Fibrinolytic inhibitors

Aminocaproic acid, BP
This inhibits the activation of plasminogen to plasmin. The relevance of endometrial fibrinolysis to menorrhagia secondary to the presence of an intra-uterine contraceptive device (IUD) was suggested by finding high fibrinolytic activity around the IUDs removed from women with excessive bleeding, and aminocaproic acid has been recommended for patients with IUDs and excessive menstrual bleeding.

Presentation

Sachets	aminocaproic acid 3 g
Syrup	aminocaproic acid 300 mg/ml in 250 ml bottle

Dose
An oral dose of aminocaproic acid 3 g should be dissolved in a glass of cold water and taken four-to-six times daily, or the syrup 10 ml should be taken a similar number of times a day.

Contraindications
The dose should be reduced in the presence of impaired renal function.

Indications
It is advised for the control of dysfunctional uterine bleeding, e.g. secondary to the presence of an IUD.

Side effects
These include dizziness, nausea, diarrhoea and hypotension. A rare but severe complication is generalized muscle pain due to an acute myopathy, with secondary renal impairment consequent on myoglobinuria.

Special features
It is also used to control excessive fibrinolytic activity in, for example, patients suffering from severe post-partum haemorrhage. It is not available in the UK.

Tranexamic acid

This is an antifibrinolytic agent which competitively inhibits the activation of plasminogen to plasmin.

Presentation

Syrup	500 mg/5 ml
Tablets	500 mg
Ampoules	100g/ ml

Dose

An oral dose of two-to-three tablets or syrup 10–15 ml, three or four times a day for 3–4 days, starting after heavy bleeding has begun.

Contraindications

Patients with a history of thromboembolic disease.

Side effects

Nausea, vomiting and diarrhoea. Giddiness may occur after intravenous use.

Special features

The dose should be reduced for patients with renal insufficiency. A 50% reduction in blood loss is normally achieved. It does not affect the histological finding at curettage. It is not available in the United States.

Hormones

There is a list of hormones now advocated for the management of dysfunctional uterine bleeding ranging from norethisterone to gonadotrophin-releasing hormones. Reported side effects (see Table 5.2) may help in choice of initial agent.

Norethisterone, BP (norethindrone, USP)

These are specifically advised in metropathia haemorrhagia and other variants of dysfunctional uterine bleeding. They induce secretory changes in oestrogen-primed proliferative endometrium.

Presentation

Tablets	5 mg
Injection	5 mg

Dose

For metropathia haemorrhagia, 5 mg should be taken three times a day for 10 days from day 5 of the cycle. For dysfunctional uterine bleeding, 5 mg should be taken twice a day or three times a day from day 19 to day 26 of the cycle (counting day 1 as the first day of menstruation) or 5–10 mg given by deep vein injection for 5–10 days until 20 days before expected menstruation.

Table 5.2 Side effects of currently used hormonal agents

Medroxyprogesterone acetate	Percentage	Danazol	Percentage	GnRH-A	Gestrinone	Percentage
Amenorrhoea	70%	Weight gain	85%	Hot flushes	Acne	48%
Dysfunctional bleeding	20%	Decreased breast size	48%	Decreased libido	Seborrhoea	48%
Cyclic bleeding	10%	Muscle cramps	52%	Vaginal dryness	Leg pain	16%
Weight gain	60%	Flushing	42%	Decreased bone mineral content	Cramps	16%
Oedema, bloating	60%	Mood changes	38%		Oedema	3%
Anxiety, irritability	20%	Seborrhoea	37%		Chloasma	3%
Depression	5%	Depression	32%		Hirsutism	15%
Breast tenderness		Sweating	32%		Hoarseness	7%
		Oedema	28%		Hair loss	7%
		Change in appetite	28%		Pruritus	13%
		Acne	27%			
		Fatigue	25%			
		Hirsutism	21%			
		Decreased libido	20%			
		Nausea	17%			
		Headache	17%			
		Dizziness	10%			
		Insomnia	10%			
		Rash	8%			
		Increased libido	8%			
		Deepening voice	7%			
		Increased low-density lipoproteins				
		Decreased high-density lipoproteins				
		Increased hepatic enzymes				
		Fetal masculinization				

Reproduced from Obstetrics and Gynaecology Clinics of North America Vol 16 March 1989 p. 108 with permission.

Contraindications

Contraindicated in patients with severe disturbance of liver function; the congenital hyperbilirubinaemias; a history of idiopathic jaundice or pruritus of pregnancy, or herpes of pregnancy.

Side effects

These include nausea, exacerbations of epilepsy and migraine and cholestatic liver changes with very high doses. Side effects of currently used hormonal agents are listed in Table 5.2.

Special features

Progesterone is also available by injection and 5–10 mg by deep i.m. injection for 5–10 days until 2 days before expected menstruation is indicated. Alternatively, medroxyprogesterone acetate 2.5–10 mg daily may be used. The pathologist should be advised that the patient has been taking the progestogen, should curettage be undertaken.

Oral contraceptives (see p. 145)

These may be used to regulate a dysfunctional uterine bleeding problem.

Danazol (see p. 66)

This hormone may be successful in regulating menorrhagia using 100 mg on alternate days throughout the menstrual cycle.

Gonadotrophin-releasing hormone agonists (see p. 66)

If used, they should be restricted to 6 months course.

Summary

Ethamsylate or tranexamic acid may be of value for patients suffering from dysfunctional bleeding secondary to an intra-uterine contraceptive device. Hormone preparations are otherwise advised in the management of patients with dysfunctional vaginal bleeding, but organic pathology must be excluded.

Further reading

Bayer, S.R. and De Cherney A.H. (1993). *Journal of the American Medical Association*, **269**(14), 1823.

Shaw, R.W. (1990). Dysfunctional uterine bleeding. *Advances in Reproductive Endocrinology*, Volume 2. Parthenon, UK.

Chapter 6

Premenstrual Syndrome

Introduction

This syndrome is characterized by the repeated appearance of one or more of a number of symptoms, normally during the week preceding menstruation. The symptoms most commonly embraced are severe headaches (often menstrual rather than premenstrual), emotional psychic states (irritability, depression, anxiety), breast tension and pain, oedema, tachycardia and digestive disturbances. Other symptoms which have been demonstrated as part of the syndrome include rhinorrhoea, exacerbation of rheumatism, nausea and vertigo, skin eruptions and mucosal lesions, but these latter symptoms appear unrelated to cyclical hormone influence.

The syndrome is extremely common and affects approximately 60% of all females, with psychic tensions as a marked feature varying from a mild form to marked states of anxiety or depression. It has been stated that the bulk of all female crime, suicide attempts and admissions to psychiatric institutions occurs during the premenstrual phase.

The aetiology of the premenstrual syndrome remains in doubt, as evidenced by the multitude of therapeutic agents administered in its management. Some of the symptoms such as breast pain and oedema, together with the cyclical nature and tendency to recur at the premenopausal stage, are suggestive of an endocrine disturbance.

The syndrome appears to be more prevalent, possibly because in earlier years other gynaecological conditions merited more detailed study. Some such conditions, including dysmenorrhoea or climacteric symptoms, are now manageable and women are describing their premenstrual symptoms in greater detail and hoping for medical therapy. Many women will suffer in silence and accept the symptomatology and, while the aetiology remains obscure, therapy is basically reassurance and support by the medical practitioner and the patient's family, with a trial of medical therapy.

Alternative therapy available includes hormonal treatment using progestogens, the combined oestrogen–progestogens or danazol, while non-hormonal therapy using pyridoxine, antispasmodics, antidepressants or diuretics have been used. Evening primrose has also been advocated. Each, and all, preparations have their advocates.

Hormone therapy

Progestogens

These have been described previously and include dydrogesterone (see p. 61) and norethisterone (see p. 61). Pure progesterone also has its advocates in preference to oral synthetic progestogens.

Progesterone, BP, Eur.P, USP

Presentation

Injections	25 mg, 50 mg, 100 mg
Implants	100 mg
Suppositories	200 mg, 400 mg

Dose

Injection: 10–20 mg to be given by intramuscular injection for the last 2 weeks of the cycle.
Implants: 2–5 of the 100 mg implants should be used every 8 months.
Suppositories/pessaries: 200–400 mg/day should be used from day 14 until the day of menstruation.

Side effects

None known.

Special feature

Nil specific.

Oestrogens (see Chapter 7)

These have also been advocated in the management of premenstrual syndrome e.g. transdermal oestradiol preparations.

Oestrogen–progestogen combinations (see p. 145)

Danazol (see p. 66)

Many patients taking danazol in the management of menorrhagia, using doses as low as 100 mg on alternate days throughout the menstrual cycle, have spontaneously volunteered an improvement in their premenstrual symptoms.

Non-hormonal therapy

Antispasmodics: hyoscine-N-butyl bromide (see p. 63)

Antidepressants

Mianserin hydrochloride
This is a tetracyclic antidepressant.

Presentation
Tablets 10 mg, 20 mg, 30 mg.

Dose
Initially an oral dose of 30–40 mg daily in divided doses or as a single dose at night, may be increased as necessary (gradually) to max of 90 mg daily.

Contraindications
Mania and severe liver disease.

Indications
It is an antidepressant.

Side effects
Drowsiness, reversible bone-marrow depression, jaundice, hypomania and convulsions, gynaecomastia, nipple tenderness and non-puerperal lactation, dizziness, postural hypotension, polyarthropathy, skin rash, sweating and tremor have all been reported on occasion. Mianserin hydrochloride may potentiate the central nervous depressant action of alcohol.

Special features
Care should be exercised in patients who have had a recent myocardial infarction or heart block. The drug should be avoided in patients with epilepsy and the dose of any concurrent therapy reviewed in patients with diabetes, hepatic or renal insufficiency, narrow-angle glaucoma and patients receiving anticoagulants or antihypertensive therapy.

If surgery is indicated, the anaesthetist should be informed of the treatment being given. It is not available in the United States.

Antiprostaglandins: mefenamic acid, BP (see p. 63)

Diuretics

Of the available diuretics, spironolactone has been recommended on the suggested evidence of aldosterone having an aetiological role.

Spironolactone, BP, USP

Presentation
Tablets 25 mg, 100 mg.

Dose
An oral dose of 100 mg per day.

Contraindications
Hypersensitivity to spironolactone or patients with hyperkalaemia.

Side effects
Potentiation of antihypertensive drugs may occur; gastrointestinal intolerance, drowsiness, headache and mental confusion may occur.

Special features
None known.

Vitamins

Pyridoxine hydrochloride, BP, Eur.P, USP (vitamin B_6)
The successful use of pyridoxine hydrochloride in the treatment of depression in oral contraceptive users and menopausal women on oestrogen replacement therapy, suggested an indication for its use in the premenstrual syndrome. There is a greatly increased need for pyridoxine hydrochloride, due to oestrogen effects on tryptophan metabolism.

Presentation
Tablets 10 mg, 20 mg, 50 mg, 100 mg.

Dose
An oral dose of 100 mg daily.

Contraindications
None known.

Side effects
None known.

Special features
None known.

Tranquillizers, e.g. diazepam (see p. 137)

Choice of preparation

The multiplicity of available preparations, with specific claims made for each, would be in accord with the failure to understand the aetiology of the syndrome. Each available preparation may be acting as a placebo, and specific benefit may be obtained by appropriate care and consideration from the patient's family, without any drug treatment. Many patients prefer herbal medications including evening primrose preparation.

Further reading

Consumers' Association (1992). Managing the Premenstrual syndrome. *Drug and Therapeutic Bulletin*, **30**(18).

O'Brien P.M.S. (1993). Helping women with premenstrual syndrome. *British Medical Journal*, **307**, 1471–1475.

Kleijner J. (1994). Editorial "Evening Primrose Oil" *British Medical Journal* **309**, 824–825.

Chapter 7

The Climacteric and Menopause

Introduction

Much has been written on this subject, not least in the women's popular journals, with reference to hormone-replacement therapy (HRT). HRT has been favoured in the United States for many years but it has been slow to gain support in the UK and many patients who commence HRT will discontinue within 12 months for various reasons, including continued menstruation. Considerable controversial debate continues within the medical profession on the advantages and disadvantages of oestrogen replacement therapy and, if elected, the choice of preparation and route of application. It appears neither needed nor justifiable to recommend routine HRT to every post-menopausal woman, but indications include the immediate short-term use to allay distressing symptoms such as vasomotor 'hot flushes' or insomnia and alternatively the long-term use to prevent osteoporosis developing due to oestrogen loss in the post-menopausal woman. HRT also protects the cardiovascular system reducing the risk of coronary thrombosis or cerebrovascular accident.

Caution has to be practised, however, due to the now accepted association of endometrial carcinoma with exogenous oestrogens — hence the preferred oestrogen–progestogen combination preparations for routine use. If oestrogens are contraindicated, alternative preparations including clonidine hydrochloride (see p. 81) and medroxyprogesterone acetate (see p. 65) are available to control the symptoms of vasomotor instability, but explanation, advice and reassurance by the medical practitioner and the family still remain paramount.

Only 10% of patients going through the climacteric have symptoms severe enough to interfere with life-style and it is mainly this group of patients who will request appropriate treatment. The climacteric is the perimenopausal phase demonstrated by irregular periods, vasomotor hot flushes or flashes, and elevated follicle-stimulating hormone. The menopause is the onset of amenorrhoea from ovarian failure and post-menopausal bleeding occurring

6 months or later indicates investigations to exclude malignancy. Community menopausal clinics have been advocated with prophylaxis of osteoporosis as the main objective. A rising follicle-stimulating hormone level with early symptomatology may indicate the appropriate starting date for therapy, but patients may be upset by regular withdrawal bleeds induced by oestrogen–progestogen combination therapy and the need for pre-therapy curettage repeated at intervals later, and compliance may be less than desired (see above). Alternative non-hormonal treatment of osteoporosis has been suggested.

The use of hormonal preparations for the suppression of menopausal symptoms is a common cause of post-menopausal bleeding. Cosmetic creams may contain oestrogens, including oestrone, oestradiol and its esters, progesterone and ethisterone. Oestrogens are also used as growth promoters in veterinary medicine.

Non-hormonal preparations

Central α-agonists

Clonidine hydrochloride BP

This is a hypotensive agent designed to relieve 'hot flushes' and vasomotor symptoms.

Presentation

Tablets 25 μg.

Dose

An oral dose of 25–50 μg should be taken twice daily, rising after 2 weeks to a maximum of 75 μg twice daily if necessary.

Contraindications

These include depressive illness. Further depressive episodes have occasionally been reported in such patients.

Side effects

Those reported include sedation, dry mouth, dizziness, nausea and nocturnal unrest. Hypertension on sudden withdrawal may also occur.

Special features

This drug is also available in a dose of 100 μg and 300 μg as Catapres (Boehringer Ingelheim) in the UK and United States where it is used for all grades of hypertension.

Minor tranquillizers, (e.g. diazepam and chlordiazepoxide) (see p. 106)

Bone regulators

Bone-density studies will give a guide as to whether therapy is indicated.

Etidronate disodium

This is now indicated in the treatment of established vertebral osteoporosis. It inhibits osteoclast activity and the dissolution of calcium hydroxyapatite crystals. It increases vertebral bone mass and reduces the rate of fresh fractures in patients presenting with severe osteoporosis and multiple fractures.

Presentation

Tablets	400 mg (di sodium etidronate)
	1.25 g (calcium carbonate)

Dose

One 400 mg dose of etidronate disodium daily in the middle of a 4-hour fast for 14 days, followed by one calcium carbonate 1,250 mg tablet daily in water for 76 days. The 90-day cycle is repeated for 3 years.

Contraindications

Severe renal impairment.

Side effects

Enterocolitis; nausea.

Special features

Discontinue if fractures occur. Monitor renal function. Maintain adequate calcium and vitamin D intake.

Salcatonin BP

This is a hormone (synthetic calcitonin) and is indicated for post-menopausal osteoporosis. It maintains bone mass by suppressing bone resorption. It is thought to inhibit the calcium pump that transports calcium from bone cells into the extracellular space.

Presentation

Injection	100 IU/ml
	200 IU/ml

Dose

100 IU daily by subcutaneous or intramuscular injection together with 600 mg elemental calcium and 400 units of vitamin D daily.

Contraindications

Nil specific.

Side effects
Nausea, vomiting, flushes, tingling hands, unpleasant taste, allergic reaction.

Special features
Interacts with cardiac glycosides. Use with caution with a history of allergy.

Calcium supplements
Many are available and calcium is readily absorbed from the gut either as gluconate, carbonate or bone extract. Supplements are indicated if the dietary intake of calcium is less than 1500 mg.

Presentation

Calcium carbonate tablets	1.25 gm (= 12.5 mmol calcium). Not available in the UK)

Dose
One-to-three daily in water.

Contraindications
Hypercalcaemia.

Side effects
Nausea, vomiting, constipation.

Special features
Use with care with impaired renal function or history of renal stones.

Hormonal therapy

Oestrogens are available either as local preparations — creams, vaginal tablets, vaginal rings — for atrophic vaginitis or as general agents — tablets, plasters, implants, — for replacement therapy. Where oestrogens are contraindicated, medroxyprogesterone acetate alone has been advocated (see p. 65).

Local atrophic vaginitis

Conjugated oestrogens, USP (Premarin; Ayerst)

Presentation
Cream; conjugated oestrogens 0.625 mg/g in a non-liquefying base, 42.5 g.

Dose
A daily dose of 2–4 g, using calibrated applicator.

Contraindications
These include neoplasms of the uterus, vagina, vulva or breast.

Indications

It is indicated for atrophic vaginitis. It may also be used vaginally prior to pelvic-floor surgery in the post-menopausal patient.

Side effects

Uterine bleeding may rarely occur.

Special features

Due to the low bulk of each application, there is little likelihood of leakage. The formula of Premarin is as follows:

Oestrone	22%
Equilin	28%
α-Dihydroequilin	11.7%
β-Dihydroequilin	1.3%
α-Oestradiol	1.8%
β-Oestradiol	0.2%

Dienoestrol, BP, Eur.P

Presentation

Cream 78 g, with applicator.

Dose

A daily dose of one-to-two full applicators should be used for up to 2 weeks and then half the dosage for a further 2 weeks. Maintenance dosage = 1 applicatorful 1 to 3 times a week after restoration of vaginal mucosa.

Contraindications

Genital-tract malignancy and breast cancer.

Indications

It is indicated for atrophic vaginitis. It may also be used vaginally prior to pelvic-floor surgery in the post-menopausal patient.

Side effects

Uterine bleeding may rarely occur.

Special features

Systemic oestrogens may also be used for atrophic vaginitis, e.g. ethinyloestradiol 10–50 μg daily for 21 days, with a 7-day interval prior to repeating the course. Vaginal creams are absorbed and act systemically.

Oestriol USP

Presentation

Tablets	0.25 mg
Cream	0.1%, 0.01%
Pessaries	0.5 mg

Dose
0.5–3 mg tablets daily for up to 30 days then 0.5–1 mg daily, or one applicatorful of cream intravaginally daily for 3 weeks then one dose twice a week.

Contraindications
As for dienoestrol.

Side effects
As for dienoestrol.

Special features
Oestradiol 25 μg pessaries are also available.

General hormone-replacement therapy

Many preparations are available, including oestrogen implants, transdermal patches or oral preparations or percutaneous creams.

Implants

Normally oestradiol would be used, but testosterone (50 mg–100 mg every 4–8 months) may be used in addition: advocates suggest this improves libido but their prolonged use is costly and usually irrational.

Oestradiol implants
These will preserve premenstrual levels of oestrogen for over 12 months. They may be used to reduce the sudden withdrawal symptoms during a routine hysterectomy and bilateral salpingo-oophorectomy (unless the operation has been performed for cancer).

Presentation

Implants	Oestradiol BPC 1968 25 mg, 50 mg, 100 mg.

Dose
Castration (with uterus); 50 mg should be used, with an expected duration of 32–36 weeks. Castration (without uterus); 50–100 mg should be used, with an expected duration of 44–52 weeks. Menopause: 50 mg should be used, with an expected duration of 32 weeks.

Contraindications

The presence of oestrogen-dependent tumours. Cardiovascular and cerebrovascular disorders, thromboembolism or history of moderate/severe hypertension, severe liver disease or history of cholestatic jaundice, history of jaundice in pregnancy, steroid induced jaundice, Rotor Syndrome, Dubin-Johnson Syndrome, Hyperlipoproteinaemia.

Side effects

Uterine bleeding may occur.

Special features

Oestradiol implants may be inserted using local anaesthetic in the clinic. Tachyphylaxis can occur and patients may request more infrequent implants of every 3–6 months; serial monitoring of serum oestradiol levels is advisable.

Transdermal preparations

Oestradiol

This is available as a transdermal patch containing 25, 50 and 100 μg. The patch is changed every 3–4 days using a different site. It is also available as a combined patch with norethisterone acetate 250 μg. The oestradiol 50 μg patch can also be used alone for 2 weeks and then coupled with norethisterone acetate 1 mg for days 15 to 26 of each 28 days of oestrogen replacement.

Oral preparations

These are used to prevent or relieve the symptoms of nocturnal sweating, nervousness, insomnia, depression, headaches and 'hot flushes', but they should be used with care in patients with thrombotic disease.

Single preparations (see Table 7.1)

These include the following tablets:

1. Piperazine oestrone sulphate 1.5 mg
2. Premarin (Ayerst), containing natural conjugated oestrogens 0.625 mg, 1.25 mg.
3. Oestradiol valerate 1 mg, 2 mg.

Each preparation has its own advocate, but oestradiol valerate will be described in further detail.

Table 7.1 Oral and transdermal preparations

Type	Oestrogen	Progestogen	Formulation
Combined			
Oestradiol/	1 mg	–	16 tablets
norethisterone	1 mg	1 mg	12 tablets
	50 μg/24 h	–	4 patches
	50 μg/24 h	250 μg/24 h	4 patches
	50μg/24 h	–	8 patches
		1mg	12 tablets (days 15–26)
Oestradiol/	1 mg	–	11 tablets
levonorgestrel	1 mg	0.25 mg	10 tablets
	2 mg	–	16 tablets
	2 mg	75 μcg	12 tablets
Oestradiol/	2 mg	–	11 tablets
norgestrel	2 mg	0.5 mg	10 tablets
Oestrogens,	0.625 mg	–	28 tablets
conjugated		0.15mg	12 tablets (days 17–28)
	1.25 mg	–	28 tablets
		0.15 mg	12 tablets (days 17–28)
Mestranol/	12.5 μg	–	5 tablets
norethisterone	25 μg	–	8 tablets
	50 μg	–	2 tablets
	25 μg	1 mg	3 tablets
	30 μg	1.5 mg	6 tablets
	20 μg	0.75 mg	4 tablets
Oestradiol/	2 mg, 1 mg	–	12 tablets
oestriol/	2 mg, 1 mg	1 mg	10 tablets
norethisterone	1 mg, 0.5 mg	–	6 tablets
	4 mg, 2 mg	–	12 tablets
	4 mg, 2 mg	1mg	10 tablets
	1 mg, 0.5 mg	–	6 tablets

Table 7.1 Continued

Type	Oestrogen	Progestogen	Formulation
Oestrogen-only			
Oestradiol	1 mg	–	28 tablets
	2 mg	–	28 tablets
	25 μg/24 h	–	8 patches
	50 μg/24 h	–	8 patches
	100 μg/24 h	–	8 patches
	1 mg	–	21 tablets
	2 mg	–	21 tablets
	2 mg	–	28 tablets
Oestrogens, conjugated	0.625 mg	–	28 tablets
	1.25 mg	–	28 tablets
Oestrone	1.5 mg	–	tablets
Oestriol/oestrone/oestradiol	0.27 mg, 1.4 mg 0.6 mg	–	tablets

Many different formulations both in the UK, USA and worldwide are available; progestogens are required as an adjunct to oestrogen replacement therapy in non hysterectomised women to protect against endometrial cancer. Tibolone 2.5 mg (Organon) – a synthetic steroid is also available and does not appear to stimulate the endometrium in women who have not menstruated in the preceding 12 months thus reducing the incidence of breakthrough bleeding, a common cause for discontinuing therapy with many women.

Oestradiol valerate (estradiol valerate, USP)

Presentation

Tablets 1 mg, 2 mg.

Dose

A daily dose of 2 mg should be taken for 21 days, followed by a 7-day interval before the next course.

Maintenance treatment.

When a satisfactory therapeutic result has been achieved, 1 mg should be taken daily for 21 days with a 7-day interval before the next course. At this dosage, longer courses of treatment are generally possible without provoking endometrial bleeding, but it is recommended that these be no longer than 6 weeks (i.e. two packs) and then the full interval of 1 week follows each course.

Contraindications
These include carcinoma of the breast or uterus, myomatous uterus, endometriosis or acute and severe chronic liver disease, jaundice and a history of idiopathic jaundice in pregnancy or severe pruritus of pregnancy. The congenital hyperbilirubinaemia syndromes are also contraindications and others include: previous or existing thrombotic processes (including cerebrovascular accident), sickle-cell anaemia, otosclerosis with deterioration in a previous pregnancy and a history of herpes of pregnancy. Severe liver function disturbances. Dubin Johnson and Rotor Syndromes. History of thromboembotic processes.

Side effects
Nausea, headache and bloating (which are largely due to water retention), hypertension, cholestasis and cholelithiasis and vaginal bleeding have all been reported. Given cyclically so as to minimize the risk of overstimulation of the endometrium, which can lead to post-menopausal bleeding. Synthetic oestrogens may carry thrombogenic hazards.

Special features
Patients receiving long-term HRT should have periodical gynaecological follow-up examination. In patients with mild chronic liver disease, the liver function should be assessed every 8–12 weeks. Patients who are still menstruating but suffering from climacteric disorders, are best treated with a cyclical oestrogen–progestogen combination. Combined oestrogen–progestogen therapy is also advocated to reduce the incidence of endometrial hyperstimulation and carcinoma, and most preparations available are listed in Table 7.1, but newer preparations are marketed at regular intervals.

Choice of preparation

The clinician should choose any of the combination preparations and become fully conversant with the chosen drug. Should the patient not have a uterus, a single oestrogen preparation may be used, otherwise a combined oestrogen–progestogen preparation is mandatory.

The therapy should be commenced as soon as there is clinical evidence of the climacteric, i.e. 'hot flushes' and insomnia, together with an elevated follicle-stimulating hormone level (>15 units). Some patients may elect to remain on the low-oestrogen oral contraceptive until there is evidence of the menopause and then continue on hormone-replacement therapy throughout life. However, for various reasons including breakthrough bleeding, only 4% of patients remain on hormone therapy after 12 months, relying on a good diet, exercise and no smoking for a healthy lifestyle.

Therapy should be continued for 18–24 months or continuously if cardiovascular accidents or osteoporosis are to be prevented, but many patients elect to accept therapy only for a short time to relieve the distressing vasomotor symptoms. The value of a sensible lifestyle with good nutrition, exercise and no smoking may be preferred by many patients.

Further reading

Martin, K.A. and Freeman, M.W. (1993). Postmenopausal Hormone Replacement Therapy. Editorial. *New England Journal of Medicine,* **328**(15).

Storm, T. *et al.* (1990). Effect of intermittent cyclical etidronate therapy on bone mass and fracture rate in women with postmenopausal osteoporosis. *New England Journal of Medicine,* **322** 1265–1271.

Studd, J.W.W. and M. Whitehouse, (1988). *The Menopause.* Blackwell Scientific Publications, Oxford, pp. 76–84.

Studd, J.W.W. (1992). Complications of hormone replacement therapy in postmenopausal women. *Journal of the Royal Society of Medicine,* **85**, 376–378.

Studd, J.W.W. and Smith R.N.J. (1994). Oestrogens and depression in women; menopause. *Journal of the North American Menopause Society,* **1**(1), 33–37.

Versi, E. and Cardozo L. (1988). Oestrogens and lower urinary tract function, in *The Menopause* (ed. J.W.W. Studd), Blackwell Scientific Publications, Oxford, pp. 76–84.

Watts, N.B. *et al.* (1990). Intermittent cyclical etidronate treatment of postmenopausal osteoporosis. *New England Journal of Medicine,* **373**, 73–79.

Chapter 8

Pain Relief and Sedatives

Introduction

The control of pain in those patients suffering from terminal cancer, for patients with chronic debilitating disease, for obstetric analgesia and for post-operative surgical procedures, has aroused concern in the lay public. Post-operative pain has generally been neglected because it is short-lived and is usually dealt with by junior staff. Analgesic requirements may be profoundly affected by the attitude of both the patient and the prescriber, but analgesics of adequate potency and dosage should be given *before* the discomfort becomes intolerable and patient-controlled syringes containing analgesics have been used with modest success in the management of post-operative pain and also during labour — this particularly applies to terminal care therapy (see p. 69).

The management of pain relief remains complex and is not necessarily restricted to drug usage.

Premedication drugs

Atropine sulphate, BP, Eur.P, USP

This anticholinergic drug, intended to reduce secretions and protect against vagal stimulation, should be given intravenously 5 minutes before surgery.

Presentation

Ampoules Normally 600 µg/ml, for injection.

Dose

An intravenous dose of 0.5–0.6 mg; 1.2 mg is given before neostigmine methylsulphate BP reversal of muscle-relaxant effects.

Side effects

Gastro-oesophageal reflux; maternal tachycardia.

Special features
May be accompanied by intravenous metoclopramide 10 mg to prevent gastro-oesophageal reflux.

Hyoscine hydrobromide, BP, USP (scopolamini hydrobromidum, Eur.P)
This has similar peripheral parasympatholytic actions to atropine sulphate, and also has a central sedative and amnesic action.

Presentation
Ampoules 0.4 mg/ml, 0.6 mg/ml.

Side effects
Bradycardia may be noted.

Special features
The drug is very mild and of no value if insomnia is due to related pain when analgesics are indicated. Use with caution in the elderly and in patients with hereditory acute porphyria (screen relatives).

Local analgesia and anaesthesia

Local anaesthetics are used to provide regional analgesia (lumbar epidural and caudal analgesia) and as local anaesthesia for minor and major surgery.

Drugs available include lignocaine hydrochloride, bupivacaine hydrochloride and, in the United States, etidocaine hydrochloride. Lignocaine is mainly used for local anaesthesia, while bupivacaine acts longer and is of specific value in epidural analgesia.

Lignocaine hydrochloride, BP (lidocaine hydrochloride, Eur.P, USP)
Lignocaine has a very rapid onset of action and a high degree of tissue penetration. Analgesia develops within 1–2 minutes and lasts for about 45 minutes with the plain solution, but may be prolonged to 1½–2 hours by the addition of a vasoconstrictor.

Presentation
Injection 0.5%, 1%, 1.5%, 2%, with or without adrenaline, in an amount not exceeding 1:200,000; 5% in 5% dextrose has been used for spinal anaesthesia.

Dose
The total dose by infiltration should not exceed 200 mg or 500 mg when given with adrenaline maximum dose 500 mg, and for lumbar epidural analgesia a 5 ml test dose of lignocaine 2% with adrenaline 1:200,000 is followed by a further 5–7 ml; 'top-up' doses of 5–10 ml are required.

Contraindications
Known hypersensitivity to local analgesics (but hypersensitivity or allergy to the amide local anaesthetics is exceedingly rare); complete heart block. Give cautiously to patients with epilepsy, impaired cardiac condition or liver damage. Also in hypovolaemia, do not use a solution containing adrenaline for anaesthesia.

Side effects
Maximum blood concentrations are reached 10–25 minutes after infiltration. The main toxic effects relate to overdose and result in excitation of the central nervous system with yawning, restlessness, excitement, nervousness, dizziness, blurred vision, nausea and vomiting, muscle twitching and convulsions. Depression with drowsiness, respiratory failure and coma may follow. Depression of the cardiovascular system with pallor, sweating, hypotension, arrhythmia and cardiac arrest may occur.

Bupivacaine hydrochloride, BP (see below)

Etidocaine hydrochloride
This is an amide local anaesthetic more potent than lignocaine, with a similarly rapid onset and a longer duration of action: it is not available in the UK.

Presentation
Injection 0.25–1.5% solutions, usually with adrenaline 1:200,000.

Dose
A 1% solution is recommended for epidural blocks for caesarean section.

Special features
Etidocaine hydrochloride has a sedative effect. It preferentially blocks motor fibres being advantageous for abdominal surgery, but may provide a satisfactory sensory block in cases where bupivacaine hydrochloride has not proved satisfactory.

Regional analgesia

Bupivacaine hydrochloride, BP

Presentation

Injection	0.5% plain or with adrenaline 1:200,000
	0.25% plain or with adrenaline 1:200,000
	0.75% plain

Dose

The dose will be advised by the anaesthetist and will normally be 4 ml for each 'top-up' as a test dose and, if no severe hypotension occurs, then a further 6 ml may be given. The maximum recommended dose in any 4-hour period is 2 mg/kg body weight representing 25–30 ml of a 0.5% solution of bupivacaine hydrochloride for a 65–70 kg adult.

Contraindications

Known sensitivity to local analgesics and complete heart block.

Side effects

Depression of the cardiovascular system with pallor, sweating, hypotension (which can be corrected with 10–50 mg intravenous ephedrine), arrhythmia and cardiac arrest may occur. A test dose of bupivacaine hydrochloride is thus mandatory, since rarely the epidural catheter may become displaced. Overdosage may result in excitation of the central nervous system with yawning, restlessness, excitement, nervousness, dizziness, blurred vision, nausea and vomiting, and respiratory failure and coma.

Special features

Epidural 'top-ups' are rarely given for more than 48 hours post-operatively, but further analgesia can be provided using parenteral narcotics. Bupivacaine hydrochloride should not be used for intravenous regional analgesia.

Parenteral analgesia

Morphine sulphate, BP, USP

This drug is more effective than pethidine hydrochloride, has a longer duration of action, but has no atropine-like antispasmodic effect and is associated with more nausea and vomiting. The central analgesic effect is enhanced by a sedative action and by mental detachment. A long-acting preparation is also available (continuous morphine sulphate).

Presentation

Injection	10 mg/ml, 15 mg/ml, 20 mg/ml, 30 mg/ml
Tablets	10 mg, 15 mg, 30 mg, 60 mg, 100 mg, 200 mg sustained release (SR)
Rectal suppositories	15 mg, 30 mg
Suspension	10 mg, 30 mg
Continuous morphine sulphate	10 mg, 30 mg (see p. 97)

Dose

An oral dose of 10–20 mg every 3–6 hours, as required, for 24 hours; or 30 mg (SR) every 12 hours for chronic pain or terminal conditions. (See Table 8.1).

Contraindications

Bronchitis and emphysema or asthma. Alcoholics and patients with convulsive disorders may be particularly sensitive to morphine. Patients taking monoamine oxidase inhibitors may react with excitation, delirium, convulsions, hyperpyrexia, respiratory depression and severe hypertension with cerebrovascular accidents.

Side effects

Euphoria and nausea and vomiting, respiratory and cough depression, constipation and tendency to dependence are common. Hypotension, urinary retention and potentiation of the action of phenothiazines have all been reported.

Special features

This is the most generally useful post-operative analgesic, but other analgesics are available including diamorphine hydrochloride (see p. 96) (not available in the United States), dextromoramide (see p. 97), Diconal (dipipanone 10 mg with cyclizine 30 mg) (see p. 97).

Pethidine hydrochloride, BP, Eur.P (meperidine hydrochloride, USP)

This is a powerful analgesic and atropine-like antispasmodic. It is relatively short acting and has a small soporific effect. It is used with diazepam in minor surgical procedures (see p. 136) and routinely for post-operative analgesia.

Presentation

Injection	50 mg/ml, 1 ml and 2 ml ampoules
Tablets	25–50 mg

Dose

1.5 mg/kg body weight intramuscularly or 100 mg orally may be given as required, but the need for repetition should be reviewed after 48 hours. Pethidine is a drug of addiction, and if the patient requests further doses after a period of 48 or 72 hours then dependency or abuse potential should be considered.

Contraindications

These include the use of monoamine oxidase inhibitors, since reactions with excitation, delirium, convulsions, hyperpyrexia, hypertension and respiratory depression have been recorded. Liver disease and biliary colic are contraindications as are patients with raised intracranial pressure, depressed respiration or obstructive airways disease.

Side effects
Nausea, vomiting, euphoria, dizziness, hypotension, respiratory depression, cough suppression, constipation, urinary retention and potentiation of the action of phenothiazines have all been reported.

Special features
Self-controlled intermittent intravenous injections of pethidine have been used by patients for relief from post-operative pain. Initial post-operative analgesia tends to be provided by intermittent parenteral analgesia given routinely on prescription 'as required every 3-4 hours'; consideration should be given to the use of patient-controlled injection using pre-loaded mechanical syringes attached to an intravenous catheter.

Pentazocine hydrochloride, BP
This is an alternative analgesic and is intermediate between pethidine and codeine in analgesic effectiveness.

Presentation

Injection	30 mg/ml, 60 mg/2 ml
Tablets	25 mg
Capsules	50 mg
Suppositories	50 mg

Dose
An oral dose of 25–100 mg every 3–4 hours or by injection 30–60 mg every 3–4 hours. Rectal suppositories 50 mg may be used up to 4 times a day.

Contraindications
Pentazocine hydrochloride may produce withdrawal symptoms in narcotic addicts; it should be used with care in patients with impaired renal or hepatic function and avoided after a myocardial infarction.

Side effects
An Lysergic-acid diethylamine (LSD)-type effect with hallucinations; nausea, vertigo, vomiting, skin flushes and visual disturbance may all occur.

Special features
Pentazocine is a mixed agonist–antagonist and can antagonize the effects of concurrently administered narcotics: there is minimal place for this drug due to a) moderate potency b) partial antagonist properties c) hallucination potential.

Diamorphine hydrochloride, BP (heroin hydrochloride)
This is the most addictive drug of the series and is not available on prescription in the United States. It is the most effective analgesic and causes less euphoria,

Table 8.1 Conversion for continuous morphine sulphate 30mg. This is for a 12-hour cover only

Morphine sulphate	
Three doses 15 mg oral morphine sulphate	= 1 dose MST 30 mg
Diamorphine	
Three doses 10 mg diamorphine	= 1 dose MST 30 mg
Dipipanone (Diconal)	
Three doses of 10 mg dipipanone	= 1 dose MST 10 mg
Nine doses of 10 mg dipipanone (e.g. three tablets 10 mg × 3)	= 1 dose MST 30 mg
Dextromoramide (Palfium)	
Six doses (12 tablets) 5 mg dextromoramide	= 1 dose MST 30 mg
Buprenorphine (6 hours' action)	
Two doses 0.4 mg	= 1 dose MST 30 mg

sedation, nausea or constipation than morphine. When used in the acute usage situation even then these observations are questionable and when used for chronic pain relief these side effects are as prevalent as for morphine.

Presentation

Injection	5 mg, 10 mg, 30 mg
Tablets	10 mg

Dose

A dose of 5–10 mg every 4–6 hours for up to 24 hours.

Contraindications

See morphine sulphate (p. 94).

Side effects

See morphine sulphate (p. 94).

Special features

The drug should be used with care in view of its addictive properties. It is never to be used on known addicts – special Home Office permission is required.

Newer analgesic preparations

The perfect drug for the treatment of post-operative pain is not available and newer drugs are introduced at intervals. Recent introductions include meptazinol hydrochloride — an opiate antagonist which produces post–operative analgesia similar to that obtained with pethidine hydrochloride and pentazocine hydrochloride — and buprenorphine, an opiate-like partial agonist–antagonist. It has a relatively long action. Many parenteral analgesics produce vomiting and anti-emetics (see Table A.10) may be required. In other cases, respiratory depression may occur and merit an antidote such as naloxone hydrochloride.

Buprenorphine hydrochloride

Presentation
Sublingual tablets 200 µg
Injection 300 µg/ml

Dose
200–400 µg every 6–8 hours
300–600 µg by i.m. or slow i.m. every 6–8 hours

Contraindications
Pregnancy.

Side effects
May present withdrawal symptoms in patients abusing opioids. Drowsiness potentiated by other centrally active agents. Occasional significant respiratory depression.

Special features
Also for epidural use but not licensed for routine use in the UK.

Narcotic antagonist

Naloxone hydrochloride, USP

This drug is a narcotic antidote and also an antagonist to pentazocine hydrochloride. Naloxone hydrochloride itself does not have agonist activity, i.e. it does not itself induce respiratory depression.

Presentation
Injection 400 µg/1 ml.

Dose
0.8–2 mg i.v. repeated at intervals of 2–3 mins to a maximum of 10 mg. Further doses may be given by intramuscular injection after 1–2 hours if required.

Contraindications
There are no definite contraindications.

Side effects
Occasional nausea or vomiting may occur.

Special features
Naloxone hydrochloride is a clinically effective narcotic antagonist in doses which are free from pharmacological effects when given to subjects who have not been pretreated with narcotics.

Oral analgesia

Of the many available preparations (see Table 8.2), any of the following may be given.

Salicylates

Aspirin, BP, Eur.P, USP
This is a non-steroidal anti-inflammatory drug (see Table 8.2). Such drugs have analgesic, anti-inflammatory and antipyretic activity. They act by inhibiting the formation of prostaglandins, which are closely involved in pain perception and pyrexial pain, from arachidonic acid via the cyclo-oxygenase pathway.

Presentation

Tablets, BP	300 mg
Tablets, dispersible, BP	300 mg
Tablets enteric coated	300 mg
Capsules, USNF	300 mg
Suppositories, USP	65 mg, 130 mg, 162 mg, 295 mg, 325 mg, 650 mg, 1300 mg

Dose
An oral dose of 300–900 mg every 3–4 hours as required max 4 g daily; dispersible tablets should be used and oral aspirin should always be administered with fluids, preferably milk.

Contraindications
Dyspepsia, gastritis, history of gastric ulcer, haemorrhagic diathesis.

Side effects
Nausea, vomiting or gastric irritation may occur. Some allergic individuals, especially asthmatics, may exhibit hypersensitivity to aspirin with reactions including urticaria and bronchospasm. Overdoses can cause acute ulceration

Table 8.2 Oral analgesia

Non-steroidal anti-Inflammatory drugs e.g.
- Aspirin and salicylates
- Ibuprofen
- Fenoprofen*
- Flurbiprofen*
- Ketorolac trometamol*
- Mefenamic acid
- Naproxen
- Piroxicam

Paracetamol

Narcotic analgesics, e.g.
- Buprenorphine hydrochloride
- Codeine
- Dextromoramide tartrate*
- Dextropropoxyphene*
- Diamorphine hydrochloride
- Dihydrocodeine tartrate
- Dipipanone hydrochloride
- Meptazinol*
- Methadone hydrochloride
- Morphine sulphate/hydrochloride
- Nalbuphine hydrochloride
- Pentazocine hydrochloride
- Phenazocine hydrobromide

* Not available in the United States.

of the stomach, gastrostaxis or salicylism with hyperpnoea, tinnitus and sweating.

Special features
Aspirin is marketed in many forms but to reduce gastric irritation, preparations containing soluble aspirin may be preferred. Use of repeated doses can interfere with the control of coumarin anticoagulants, causing haemorrhage.

Paracetamol, BP (acetaminophen, USP)
This analgesic also has antipyretic but no anti-inflammatory actions. It is a *p*-aminophenol derivative. It is now generally preferred to aspirin, as it is much less likely to cause gastric irritation.

Presentation

Paracetamol tablets	120 mg, 325 mg, 500 mg
Paracetamol elixir	120 mg/5ml

Dose

An oral dose of up to 4 g daily in divided doses.

Contraindications

Impaired kidney or renal function. May interfere with coumarin anticoagulant control after prolonged regular use.

Side effects

Haematological reactions such as thrombocytopenia and skin eruptions have been reported. A single oral dose of 10–15 g can cause severe liver damage up to several days later, and this can be lethal. Renal failure, heart damage, generalized bleeding and hypoglycaemia are other possible consequences of overdose.

Special features

Ideally, not more than 20 tablets should be dispensed at a time and they should be stored in childproof containers out of reach of children.

Narcotic analgesics

Dextropropoxyphene hydrochloride, BP (propoxyphene hydrochloride, USP)

This is an analgesic related to methadone hydrochloride, with an onset and duration of action similar to that of codeine, but with a slightly less potent effect. Narcotic analgesics act on specific receptors within the CNS to relieve pain, which are part of the body's own pain-regulating system which involves the enkephalins and endorphins.

Presentation

Dextropropoxyphene capsules, BP	65 mg, 150 mg
Propoxyphene hydrochloride capsules, USP	32 mg, 65 mg
Propoxyphene napsylate oral suspension, USNF	50 mg/5 ml
Propoxyphene napsylate tablets, USNF	100 mg

Dose

An oral dose of up to 260 mg daily in divided doses; 32–65 mg every 6 hours.

Contraindications

Respiratory depression; bronchial asthma. Should not be given to patients taking monoamine oxidase inhibitors.

Side effects
Dizziness, drowsiness, nausea and vomiting are the commonest.

Special features
High doses (greater than 720 mg/day) may have a toxic convulsant action. This effect of dextropropoxyphene hydrochloride may be enhanced by central nervous system stimulants such as amphetamine, occurring with lower dextropropoxyphene doses. Dextropropoxyphene has a low liability to produce dependence. Many proprietary preparations are available. The USP and USNF preparations are not available in the UK.

Dihydrocodeine tartrate, BP
This has analgesic properties, and like all narcotics tends to suppress coughing and to cause constipation. If it is used for post-operative patients, active physiotherapy to promote coughing should be instituted and laxatives used if necessary.

Presentation

Tablets	30 mg
Elixir	10 mg/5 ml
Injection	50 mg/ml

Dose
An oral dose of 30–60 mg every 4–6 hours as required, or an intramuscular/subcutaneous injection, of up to 50 mg, every 4–6 hours as required.

Contraindications
Similar to those of morphine sulphate (see p. 94).

Side effects
Similar to those of morphine sulphate (see p. 94), but side effects from dihydrocodeine tartrate are less pronounced.

Special features
Preparations containing dihydrocodeine tartrate with aspirin or paracetamol are also available. Does not cause spasm of sphincter of oddi and orally 30 mg = 100 mg oral Pethidine.

Inhalational analgesia

For post-operative physiotherapy, or for a change of dressings, the self-administration of oxygen and nitrous oxide can be invaluable. Other inhalational analgesics include trichloroethylene and methoxyflurane.

Nitrous oxide, BP, Eur.P, USP

This is pre-mixed with oxygen in equal volumes and dispensed in blue and white cylinders. It is used for inhalations from a machine, controlled by the patient. Machines are also available which allow a controlled concentration of nitrous oxide in oxygen to be given, but no more than 70% nitrous oxide should be used.

Dose

Inhalation is continued until analgesia is obtained. It takes 20 seconds or so to work and the effect is at a maximum after 45–60 seconds.

Contraindications

None known.

Side effects

Nausea and vomiting may occur. Occasionally, confusion and loss of cooperation results from the use of 70% nitrous oxide.

Special features

Entonox cylinders must be stored horizontally for 24 hours at a temperature above 10°C before use, to ensure that the constituent gases have not been exposed to cold and separated.

Trichloroethylene, BP, Eur.P

This is a volatile anaesthetic used for the production of analgesia without any loss of consciousness (0.35–0.5% mixture in air).

Presentation

A blue volatile liquid consisting of trichloroethylene with thymol 0.01% and an inert dye.

Dose

Inhalation of a 0.35–0.5% mixture in air from a Tecota Mark VI (BOC Medishield) or Emotril (BOC Medishield) vaporizer is continued until sufficient clinical analgesia is obtained.

Contraindications

History of cardiac arrhythmias; liver disease, diabetes mellitus and pre-eclampsia have been cited as contraindications, since trichloroethylene can depress liver or kidney function.

Side effects

Nausea, vomiting, drowsiness and loss of co-operation may occur. Maternal tachypnoea and tachycardia and cardiac arrhythmias may also arise and persist for many hours after trichloroethylene is discontinued.

Special features

The concurrent administration of adrenaline (for example, in association with local anaesthetics) and trichloroethylene is inadvisable, since cardiac arrhythmia may occur. The latter should be stored in cool light-proof containers in a cool place, since decomposition to phosgene and hydrochloric acid may occur.

Trichloroethylene must not be used in a closed-circuit apparatus, since heat produced by the action of carbon dioxide and water vapour on the soda lime produces dichloroacetylene which can cause cranial palsies and death. Anaesthetic machines must be checked in this respect every time trichloroethylene is used, and the reservoir should be emptied and replaced at the end of such a procedure.

Methoxyflurane, BP, USP

This agent can be used to provide analgesia or anaesthesia. It is slowly absorbed and expelled and gives prolonged analgesia.

Presentation

Methoxyflurane is a clear colourless liquid.

Dose

Methoxyflurane, 0.35% in air at all temperatures may be used for pain relief. Not more than the vapour originating from a maximum of 15 ml of the agent should be administered on any one occasion to an individual patient.

Contraindications

Liver disease.

Side effects

Nausea, vomiting, drowsiness and loss of co-operation may arise. Hypotension, respiratory depression, bradycardia and post-analgesic vomiting have all been reported, but the last is much less common than with trichloroethylene (see p. 103).

Special features

Nil specific.

Local preparations for analgesia (see Chapter 10)

Hydrocortisone acetate in many forms is used for perineal pain, e.g. following perineal surgery or for haemorrhoids (see p. 122).

Perineal bruising

Chymoral

Chymoral (Armour) contains purified proteolytic enzymes, providing trypsin and chymotrypsin activity.

Presentation

Tablets 50,000 or 10,0000 units of proteolytic activity.

Dose

An oral dose of 100,000 units four times daily, taken half an hour before meals and swallowed whole.

Contraindications

None known.

Side effects

Slight gastric disturbances may be noticed.

Bromelains

This is a mixture of proteolytic enzymes which acts directly on fibrin, depolymerizing the fibrin deposited on the tissues and in the capillary walls. By removing fibrin, it increases capillary permeability, restores drainage and reduces swelling.

Presentation

Tablets 50,000 units, 100,000 units.

Dose

An oral dose of 100,000 units four times a day.

Contraindications

Bleeding diathesis; severe hepatic or renal disease.

Special features

Anticoagulants may be potentiated.

Sedatives

Barbiturates are not now recommended due to habituation, and alternative sedatives available include chloral betaine or nitrazepam. Other benzodiazepines of use include diazepam and chlordiazepoxide hydrochloride.

Chloral betaine, BP

This is a mild sedative and is a complex of chloral with phenazone.

Presentation

Tablets	707 mg (≡ chloral hydrate 414 mg)
Elixir	143 mg/5 ml chloral hydrate

Dose

An oral dose of 1–2 tablets (15–45 ml elixir), best taken with milk.

Contraindications

Acute intermittent porphyria — chloral may precipitate an attack. Significant hepatic or renal disease or severe cardiac disease.

Nitrazepam, BP

This is similar to diazepam (see p. 137), it is mainly used for night sedation, acting in 30–60 minutes to produce sleep lasting for 6–8 hours.

Presentation

Tablets	5 mg, 10 mg
Capsules	5 mg

Dose

An oral dose of 2.5–10 mg.

Contraindications

It should be used with caution in patients with chronic obstructive lung disease or respiratory failure.

Side effects

Drowsiness or lightheadedness may occur.

Special features

Nitrazepam does not affect plasma concentration or metabolism of anticoagulants.

Diazepam, BP, USP

This is a benzodiozepine and is used as a mild tranquillizer; it also has muscle-relaxant properties and is used as a premedicant before minor surgical procedures (see p. 137). Other benzodiazepines of use include chlordiazepoxide hydrochloride and nitrazepam.

Chlordiazepoxide hydrochloride, BP, Eur.P, USP

This is used as a sedative in mild to moderate anxiety states and insomnia due to tension.

Presentation

Tablets	5 mg, 10 mg, 25 mg
Capsules	5 mg, 10 mg
Ampoules	100 mg

Dose
An oral dose of 20–100 mg daily, given after meals in divided doses; 50–100 mg may be given by intramuscular injection for acute agitation and repeated if necessary in 2–4 hours.

Contraindications
Nil specific.

Side effects
Drowsiness and ataxia may occur. Other central nervous system depressants may be summated.

Special features
Nil specific.

SUMMARY
Pain relief is complex. Following surgery, analgesics will be indicated. Post-operative regional analgesia, if used during surgery, is soon followed by parenteral or oral preparations. Self-controlled intermittent analgesic injections or inhalational analgesics are of especial value. Regional pain clinics play a major role in the management of intractable pelvic pain.

Further reading

Consumers' Association. Editorial (1993). Managing post-operative pain. *Drug and Therapeutics Bulletin*, **31**(3).

Justins, D. *et al.* (1993). Modern approaches to pain management. *Prescribers' Journal*, **33**(6).

Rowbotham, D. (1993). Postoperative pain in modern approaches to pain management. *Prescribers' Journal*, **33**(6), pgs 237–243.

Chapter 9

The Unstable Bladder

Introduction

A carefully taken history and full examination are the first essentials of management in the patient with urinary incontinence. The exclusion of any urinary-tract infection is mandatory, and pressure–flow studies may be necessary to identify the nature of the incontinence in patients with an unstable bladder. Surgery will help 95% of patients with incontinence, whereas the remainder with urinary retention (anticholinergic drugs) or frequency (antispasmodic drugs) may be helped using drugs.

The multiplicity of drugs affecting the bladder and urethra indicates no specific drug of choice. Few are potent, but specific drugs to subdue bladder irritability related to the hypertonic, unstable bladder of small capacity are available. Clinically, these are normally anticholinergic drugs, but mild tranquillizers may also be of help in the management of psychosomatic urge incontinence. For the post-menopausal patient with detrusor irritability and atrophic distal urethritis, low-dose oestrogens may also be used. Symptomatic therapy for interstitial cystitis is listed.

Anticholinergic drugs

These promote bladder voiding by increasing the tone of the detrusor muscle. They act by competing for the same drug receptors as acetylcholine.

Bethanechol chloride, USP

Presentation
Tablets 10 mg, 25 mg.

Dose
An oral dose of 10–25 mg, three or four times daily, half an hour before food.

Contraindications
Intestinal or urinary obstruction. Caution should be exercised in patients with asthma, cardiovascular disease, epilepsy, parkinsonism, vagotonia, hyperthyroidism, elderly patients, peptic ulceration, bradycardia, recent

myocardial infarction, and any condition where an increased urinary or gastrointestinal tract activity could be harmful.

Side effects

Parasympathomimetic effects such as nausea, vomiting, sweating, bradycardia and intestinal colic.

Special features

Nil specific.

Distigmine bromide

This is an anticholinesterase with maximum inhibition of plasma cholinesterase occurring 9 hours after a single intramuscular dose of 0.5 mg distigmine bromide.

Presentation

Tablets	5 mg
Injection	0.5 mg/ml

Dose

An intramuscular injection of 0.5 mg 12 hours after surgery and every 24 hours until normal function is restored, or 5 mg may be taken orally 30 minutes before breakfast until normal function is restored.

Indications

It is used in the management of patients with urinary retention following surgery.

Special features

Overdosage of the anticholinergic drugs may be counteracted by atropine (2 mg by intramuscular injection and repeated at intervals until signs of mild atropinization appear, i.e. dry mouth, mydriasis). Distigmine bromide should be used with caution in conditions where the potentiation of acetylcholine effects is undesirable, including bronchial asthma, cardiac disease, peptic ulcer, epilepsy and parkinsonism.

Neostigmine bromide, BP, Eur.P., USP

This is indicated for post-operative urinary retention.

Presentation

Tablets	15 mg
Injection	0.5 mg/ml
	2.5 mg/ml

Dose

0.5–2.5 mg intramuscularly or subcutaneously as required usual total daily dose 5–20 mg; or one to two tablets. Total daily dose 75–300 mg.

Contraindications

These include post-operative shock, serious circulatory insufficiency, serious spastic or mechanical ileus and pregnancy. It should be used with caution where doubt exists as to the integrity of any bowel anastomosis. In myasthenia gravis, where short-acting cholinergic drugs are taken concurrently, their dosage should be reduced to the minimum required to control symptoms.

Side effects

Those due to overdosage include anorexia, nausea and vomiting, abdominal cramps and diarrhoea. With the percutaneous absorption of liquid, localized sweating or muscular fasciculation are the earliest manifestations. Other effects include extreme salivation, sweating, bradycardia and hypotension GI discomfort, involuntary defecation and micturation miosis, nystagmus, agitation, excessive dreaming, weakness leading to fasciculation and paralysis..

Special features

It interacts with depolarizing muscle relaxants; cyclopropane and halothane anaesthesia.

Oxybutynin hydrochloride

This has direct antispasmodic action on the smooth muscle of the bladder detrusor as well as having anticholinergic action.

Presentation

Tablets	2.5 mg, 3 mg, 5 mg
Elixir	2.5 mg/5 ml

Dose

5 mg b.d. or t.d.s. up to a maximum of 20 mg.

Contraindications

Obstruction of bladder or gastrointestinal tract including intestinal atony, toxic megacolon, severe ulcerative colitis, myasthenia gravis, glaucoma and significant bladder outflow obstruction.

Side effects

Anticholinergic effects; facial flushing.

Special features

It interacts with phenothiazines, amantadine, butyrophenones, levodopa, digoxin and tricyclic antidepressants, and should be used with caution in patients with coronary artery disease, cardiac arrhythmias or congestive cardiac failure.

Propantheline bromide, BP, USP

This is a synthetic quaternary ammonium compound.

Presentation

Tablets 15 mg
Ampoules 30 mg/ml

Dose

An oral dose of up to 90 mg daily may be taken. (15–30 mg bd or tds one hour before meals)

Contraindications

These include glaucoma and organic pyloric stenosis.

Indications

It is advised in the management of psychosomatic urge incontinence and urinary frequency.

Side effects

Those reported include dry mouth, blurred vision, dilated pupils, lack of accomodation and light sensitivity, flushing dry skin, constipation, and mild tachycardia,

Special features

The parenteral form is not available in the UK.

Antispasmodic–musculotrophic drugs

Falvoxate hydrochloride

This is a tertiary amine chromone which selectively acts on the muscle receptor and produces muscle relaxation. It has a direct antispasmodic action on smooth-muscle fibres, and exerts its effect by increasing the local concentration of cyclic adenosine monophosphate. It is classically considered to be an antimuscarinic drug.

Presentation

Tablets 100 mg.

Dose

An oral dose of 200 mg should be taken three times a day.

Contraindications

These include patients with glaucoma, pyloric or duodenal obstruction, ileus and also obstructive uropathies of the lower urinary tract. Severe ulcerative colitis or toxic mega colon.

Indications
It is indicated for the symptomatic relief of dysuria, urgency, nocturia, vesical suprapubic pain, frequency and incontinence, and for the relief of vesico-urethral spasms due to, for example, catheterization.

Side effects
Those reported include headache, nausea, diarrhoea, blurred vision and dry mouth.

Special features
It may be used as a supplement to antibiotic therapy. It is not available in the United States.

Miscellaneous

Many other drugs are used in the management of increased bladder activity or atonicity and these include:

1. **Bromocriptine** (see p. 158) which decreases the frequency, nocturia and urgency and increases the functional bladder capacity as assessed by cystometry.
2. **Ephedrine**, which has been used in the management of enuresis secondary to involuntary detrusor contractions occurring during sound sleep.
3. **Sympathomimetic β-adrenergic stimulants**, including orciprenaline, salbutamol and terbutaline sulphate.
4. **Tricyclic antidepressants** such as imipramine, which have anticholinergic, antimuscarinic properties.
5. **Oestrogens** (see p. 83) which are of value for the post-menopausal patient with detrusor irritability and atrophic distal urethritis.
6. **Prostaglandins** and **dinoprostone** (see p. 140) which have been shown experimentally to be naturally produced by the detrusor and are used in the management of chronic retention.
7. **Vasopressin analogues — desmopressin** supplements the natural hormone and is useful for nocturnal enuresis.

Interstitial cystitus

Intra-vesical dimethyl sulfoxide (RIMSO–50, Britannia)

Interstitial cystitis (Hunner's ulcer) is a rare condition of unknown aetiology which is extremely troublesome to the patient and her gynaecologist. The main symptoms are intense suprapubic pain and urgency relieved only partially by voiding. Bladder capacity is reduced. The treatment is only symptomatic and the most efficacious treatment described is local instillation of dimethyl sulfoxide.

Pharmacology

Dimethyl sulfoxide (DMSO) is a derivative of lignin. It has good solvent properties and crosses body membranes. It has anti-inflammatory activity and in low concentrations, also causes a reversible inhibition of nerve conduction, a possible mode of its action. It also dissolves pathological deposits of collagen as in keloids. It causes a release of histamine and thus vasodilatation. It is mainly exchanged unchanged in the urine and partly via lungs.

Side effects

Garlic-like odour to the breath and skin is often observed. Urethral irritation can occur and hence lignocaine application to urethra is necessary. DMSO is known to cause changes in the refractive index of lenses in animals, but no such toxicity has been noticed in human studies. However, slit lamp studies of the eyes is recommended during treatment. Some patients initially complain of worsening of symptoms due to bladder spasm. Release of histamine can cause an hypersensitivity type reaction on occasion. Renal and hepatic damage should also be looked for, if treatment continues long term.

Contraindications

Pregnancy and lactation.

Presentation

Sterile aqueous solution of DMSO 50% w/w in bottles of 50 ml.

Dosage and administration

The urethra is anaesthetized with lignocaine jelly and 50 ml of DMSO is administered directly into the bladder with a catheter or syringe, after first emptying the bladder. It is allowed to remain inside for 15 minutes after which it can be voided. The treatment is repeated generally every 2 weeks until symptomatic relief. Generally 4–6 treatments are given. After the initial treatment, intermittent treatments are given if and when necessary. Some clinicians give an oral belladonna preparation to prevent bladder spasm in the sensitive. Others combine DMSO with corticosteroids (100 mg of hydrocortisone with 50 ml of DMSO). It has been licensed in the UK only for the purpose of bladder intallation.

SUMMARY
In the absence of obvious clinical signs, and where diagnostic difficulties pertain, bladder pressure studies are mandatory prior to medical or surgical therapy in the management of the incontinent woman.

Further reading

Robinson, T.G. and Castledon, C.M. (1994). Drugs in focus; oxybutynin hydrochloride. *Prescribers' Journal*, **34** (1), 27–30.

Chapter 10

Miscellaneous Topics

Introduction

This chapter will consider the following:

1. Anticoagulation.
2. Large bowel disorders.
3. Infusions.
4. Radiological contrast media.
5. Non-specific agents.

Anticoagulation

The management of deep venous thrombosis and potential subsequent pulmonary embolism lies in prophylaxis using subcutaneous heparin, intravenous fluids and supportive stockings. Where a thrombosis is suspected, bilateral phlebography may be needed for confirmative diagnosis.

Prophylactic therapy

The prophylaxis of deep-vein thrombosis is mainly by: physiotherapy; dieting; reduction in smoking; elective timing of surgery; intermittent calf compression during surgery; and antiplatelet drugs (aspirin).

Low-dose heparin has been specifically advocated for patients over 40 years of age or with a history of deep-vein thrombosis, who are obese or have malignant disease and are requiring major gynaecological surgery. It is not unreasonable to prescribe heparin prophylactically for all major cases. Other preparations available include dextran 70.

Antiplatelet drugs, including aspirin, and hydroxychloroquine reduce platelet adhesion and aggregation. Aspirin inhibits the formation of thromboxane A_2 by the platelets and prevents the release of pro-aggregatory ADP.

Low molecular-weight heparins neutralize Factor Xa but have proportionately less anti-IIa activity than standard heparin. They do not significantly influence platelet aggregation of binding of fibrinogen to platelets and consequently have a greater effect on thrombus formation with fewer haemorrhagic effects. It is unnecessary to monitor treatment since they do not affect blood-clotting tests.

Enoxaparin

Presentation
20 mg/0.2 ml
40 mg/0.4 ml

Dose
Single-dose pre-filled syringes.
20 mg by deep subcutaneous injection 2 hours pre-operatively and 20 mg daily for 7–10 days for moderate risk surgery; 40 mg 12 hours prior to surgery and 40 mg daily for 7–10 days for high risk surgery.

Contraindications
Acute bacterial endocarditis, major bleeding disorders, thrombocytopenia, active peptic ulcer, haemorrhagic cerebrovascular accident.

Side effects
Thrombocytopenia, liver abnormalities, haemorrhagic manifestations (bruising).

Special features
Interacts with oral anticoagulants, antiplatelet agents, non-steroidal anti-inflammatory drugs and dextran.

Sodium heparin or calcium heparin injection

Presentation
Injection 5000 units/0.2 ml.

Dose
A deep subcuticular injection of 5,000 (and 10,000 units in pregnancy) should be given every 12 hours. Treatment should begin 2 hours before surgery and continue every 8–12 hours for 5–7 days or until the patient is fully mobile.

Contraindications
These include haemophilia, purpura or other haemorrhagic states, gastric or duodenal ulcer, subacute bacterial endocarditis, advanced hepatic disease, and threatened abortion or uncontrolled hypertension.

Side effects
Febrile and allergic reactions may occur; osteoporosis may follow prolonged dosage, and also skin necrosis. Overdosage, thrombocytopenia and

haemorrhage may arise. (The heparin can be neutralized with protamine sulphate, see p. 120)

Special features

The treatment should be controlled by monitoring blood-clotting times.

Dextran 70 injection, BP

This glucose polymer is of 70,000 average molecular weight. It reduces platelet adhesiveness and has an inhibitory effect on the changes in Factors V and VIII, and fibrinogen during surgery. It has anti-sludging and antithrombotic activities similar to dextran 40 injection.

Presentation

Dextran 70 in 0.9% sodium chloride (1000 ml)
Dextran 70 in 5% dextrose (1000 ml)

Dose

500 mls over 4–6 hours during or at end of surgery then 500 ml over 4–6 hours next day. In high risk patients continue this regime on alternative days for max of 10 days.

Contraindications

It should be used with caution in patients vulnerable to vascular overloading (congestive heart failure, renal disease).

Special features

Dextran 70 and pneumatic legging have been shown to reduce the incidence of pulmonary embolism among treated patients, but not the incidence of deep-vein thrombosis.

Active therapy

Mild analgesics, physiotherapy and local heparinoid creams are used for superficial venous thrombosis. Phenylbutazone was previously used, but the hazards of associated blood dyscrasias would contraindicate this preparation.

Local heparinoid creams

These creams counteract inflammation and promote the resorption of local oedema and extravasated blood and locally delay blood clotting. Two creams are available: Lasonil (Bayer), which contains 5000 HBD units and 15,000 units hyaluronidase in 100 g, and Hirudoid (Luitpold-Werk: Farillon), which contains 25,000 units organoheparinoid of animal origin in 100 g.

Presentation

Cream	100 g
Gel	100 g
Ointment	100 g

Dose
The cream should be applied three times a day.

Contraindications
None known.

Side effects
These creams should not be applied to open wounds.

Special features
The above preparations are recommended for similar conditions, including superficial thrombophlebitis developing after intravenous injections.

Bilateral phlebography is a useful adjuvant to confirm the diagnosis of deep venous thrombosis pre-therapy.

Anticoagulants

Parenteral: Heparin, standard or low-molecular weight (see below). Standard heparin prevents coagulation by binding antithrombin-III (AT-III); this accelerates the combination of AT-III with thrombin (IIa) to form an inactive complex which is then unable to convert fibrinogen to fibrin. Heparin also neutralizes Factor Xa which prevents the conversion of prothrombin to thrombin.

Oral: These are coumarins or indanediols and act by competitively antagonizing vitamin K, indirectly inhibiting the synthesis of the plasma clotting Factors VII, IX, X and II (prothrombin). There is a latent phase (24–72 hours) before their full effect occurs and their effect may be prolonged when therapy is discontinued. Drug interactions with other plasma protein-bound drugs are common.

Heparin, BP (calcium heparin; heparin sodium, USP)
This inhibits the activation of prothrombin; it acts immediately and is given intravenously.

Presentation

Injections (vials)	1000 units/ml for therapy
	5000 units/ml for therapy
	12,500 units/ml for therapy
	25,000 units/ml for therapy
Injection (ampoules)	calcium heparin injection 5000 units (for prophylaxis)
	sodium heparin injection 5000 units (for prophylaxis)

Dose

An intravenous loading dose to 5,000 units is given (or 10,000 units if there is evidence of severe pulmonary embolism); the infusion should continue at 1000–2000 units per hour adjusted to haematological results. After 48 hours anticoagulation may be continued with warfarin sodium.

A prophylactic dose of 5000 units is given intramuscularly, twice daily, while the patient is an in-patient in hospital.

Contraindications

These include haemophilia, purpura or other haemorrhagic states, gastric or duodenal ulcer, subacute bacterial endocarditis, advanced hepatic disease, and uncontrolled hypertension.

Side effects

Those reported include febrile or allergic reactions, overdosage (bleeding can occur with either intravenous or subcutaneous administration of heparin, even with adequate laboratory control); osteoporosis and spontaneous fractures have been reported when heparin was given for 6 months or more.

Special features

Anticoagulation is a dangerous procedure which should only be undertaken in association with the haematological staff.

Management of overdosage

Heparin may be neutralized by intravenous protamine sulphate (5 ml of a 1% solution should be given in 10 minutes); 1 mg protamine neutralises 100 units heparin.

Warfarin sodium, BP, USP

The common derivatives all have similar pharmacological properties. They depress prothrombin, and also Factors VII, IX and X. Warfarin sodium antagonizes vitamin K and acts in 36–48 hours. It is monitored by measuring the prothrombin time.

Presentation

Tablets 1 mg, 3 mg 5 mg.

Dose

The initial dose is 10 mg daily for 2 days (preferably after baseline prothrombin time) Further doses are monitored according to the prothrombin time (the maintenance dose is normally 3–10 mg). A single large dose should be given initially, the size of which varies with age, body weight and degree of illness. In general, the old or very ill or very small people require smaller initial doses and younger, heavier or relatively fit people should have higher initial doses.

Contraindications

These include pregnancy.

Indications

It is used for the maintenance therapy of deep-vein thrombosis or pulmonary embolism after initial therapy with heparin.

Side effects

Those occurring include bleeding, petechiae and haematuria.

Special features

Complications of warfarin treatment suggested action below in Table 10.1.

Patients should carry 'anticoagulation cards' with them at all times, since many drugs may interact with warfarin sodium. Interactions may be due to changes in rates of hepatic removal (e.g. paracetamol) or displacement from protein binding (e.g. aspirin). Tables 10.2 and 10.3 list drugs that give a decreased response and an increased response, respectively, to warfarin sodium.

Table 10.1

Senarios	*Action*
Life threatening haemorrhage	Vit K_1, slow i.v. 5 mg and concentrate of factors II IX and X (VII conc if available or 1l of fresh frozen plasma if concs not available
Less severe haemorrhage (haematuria etc)	With hold warfarin 1 or more days, consider giving 0.5–2 mg Vit K_1, slow i.v. *High dose VIT K_1, may prevent oral anticoagulants working for several days, even weeks.*
INR4.5–7, no haemorrhage	With-hold warfarin 1–2 days, review
INR > 7, no haemorrhage	With-hold warfarin and consider 0.5 mg i.v. VIT K_1 slowly
INR in therapeutic range, haemorrhage	Always investigate e.g possible renal or GI cause

INR = International Normalized Ratio

Table 10.2 Drugs giving a decreased response to warfarin sodium

Adrenocorticosteroids
Antihistamines
Barbiturates
Chloral hydrate
Cholestyramine
Corticotrophin (ACTH)
Dichloralphenazone
Glutethimide
Griseofulvin (possibly)
Haloperidol
Meprobamate
Mercaptopurine
Methylxanthines
Oestrogens
Oral contraceptives
Phenobarbitone (and other barbiturates)
Phenytoin (may also increase anticoagulant response)
Vitamin K (and multi-vitamin preparations)

Table 10.3 Drugs giving an increased response to warfarin sodium. (This list is not exhaustive and many are clinically insignificant)

Alcohol
Allopurinol
Aluminium nicotinate
Amiodarone
Anabolic steroids (but not quinbolone)
Aspirin (and other salicylates)
Benziodarone (but not amiodarone hydrochloride)*
Bromelains*
Chloramphenicol
Cinchophen•
Clofibrate (probably)
Dextrothyroxine sodium
Diazoxide
Disulfiram
Ethacrynic acid
Glucagon
Heparin
Mefenamic acid
Methandienone*
Methylphenidate hydrochloride
Nalidixic acid
Neomycin
Norethandrolone*
Nortriptyline hydrochloride
Oxymetholone
Oxyphenbutazone
Paracetamol*
Phenylbutazone
Phenyramidol hydrochloride*
Phenytoin (may also decrease anticoagulant response)
Probenecid
Quindine
Quinine
Salicylates
Sulphamethoxazole
Sulphonylurea hypoglycaemic agents
Tetracyclines
Tolbutamide

* Not available in the United States.

Miscellaneous

Other anticoagulant therapy available includes the fibrinolytics and streptokinase or urokinase. The fibrinolytics act by stimulating the activation of endogenous plasminogens to plasmin which acts directly on fibrin, breaking it down to achieve thrombolysis. These are rarely indicated in gynaecological practice and if elected should be used with strict haematological control.

Large bowel disorders

This section relates to the treatment available for haemorrhoids, and constipation. In all cases, underlying pathology should be excluded prior to using any preparation.

Haemorrhoids — soothing agents

The basis of most preparations is an anti-inflammatory agent, for example **hydrocortisone**, or non-specific agents including **zinc oxide** and **bismuth**. If infection is present, anti-infective agents may be included but their value, other than as a placebo, must be doubtful. They may relieve pain by reducing perineal oedema and haematomata. Ultrasonic therapy may also be of value. Preparations available include:

1. Bismuth subgallate, compound suppositories, BPC — similar to Anusol (Warner), Anusol-HC containing hydrocortisone acetate and Anugesic-HC containing pramoxine hydrochloride and hydrocortisone acetate.
2. Hydrocortisone suppositories and cream — similar to Hepacort Plus (Rona Laboratories), Proctofoam HC (Stafford-Miller) and Scheriproct (Schering Chemicals).

Laxatives/enemas

Laxatives may be considered under the following classification:

1. Chemical laxatives.
2. Hydrophilic bulking agent.
3. Spasmolytics.
4. Enemata.

It should be remembered that constipation is often best treated by modifying the diet.

Chemical laxatives. Many are now obsolete or unacceptable, including liquid paraffin, dioctyl sodium sulphosuccinate (DSS) and the poloxalkols. DSS has been considered a hepatotoxin. Chemical laxatives considered suitable for special purposes include the following.

Saline laxatives

These act by maintaining a volume of fluid in the bowel by osmosis.

Presentation

Magnesium sulphate mixture, BP.

Dose

An oral dose of 5–10 ml should be taken each morning.

Indications

They are specifically advised for preparing the lower bowel for radiology.

Special features

None.

Lactulose

This synthetic disaccharide cannot be hydrolysed by the enzymes of the small intestine. It passes into the ascending colon and is split into low-molecular-weight organic acids which increase the intracolonic osmotic pressure, stimulate the colonic musculature and form a soft stool.

Presentation

Syrup

lactulose	50% w/w
lactose	5% w/w
galactose	8% w/w

Dose

15 ml bd gradually and according to patients requirements

Contraindications

These include galactosaemia.

Side effects

Those reported include intestinal bloating from gas formation.

Special features

It is not absorbed and is unlikely to adversely affect diabetics, babies or pregnant women. It may be diluted with water or fruit juice. A delay in action for 48 hours may occur and large quantities (up to 8 g or more daily) may have to be given to produce a laxative effect; the formulation can vary according to product.

Bisacodyl, BP, USP

Bisacodyl is a polyphenolic laxative, like **Phenolphthalein** (dermal sensitization and drug eruptions are well documented — phenolphthalein is therefore not recommended). Bisacodyl has no action on the small bowel and does not give rise to digestive disturbances.

Presentation

Tablets	5 mg
Suppositories	10 mg

Dose

An oral dose of one or two tablets should be taken at night. One suppository should be used in the morning.

Contraindications

Intestinal obstruction.

Side effects

Griping has been reported. Prolonged use can cause atonic non-functioning colon and hypokalaemia.

Special features

Bisacodyl is an enteric-coated tablet and should not be crushed or chewed. Antacids should not be given within 1 hour of administering the tablets. Bisacodyl is also marketed as Dulcodos (Boehringer Ingelheim), which is bisacodyl 5 mg, dioctyl sodium sulphosuccinate (DSS) 100 mg — it is not recommended since DSS is considered hepatotoxic.

Senna fruit, BP, Eur.P

Besides Senna, this group includes cascara, frangula bark, aloes and rhubarb. The active ingredients are anthraquinones which are absorbed into the bloodstream and act on the muscle of the large bowel 8–12 hours later.

Senna tablets contain sennosides A and B equivalent to sennoside B, 7.5 mg.

Presentation

Tablets	sennoside B, 7.5 mg
Granules	5ml spoonful = total sennoside B, 15 mg/5 ml
Syrup	5ml = total sennoside B, 7.5 mg/5 ml

Dose

Tablets: Two-to-four should be taken at night. Granules: 2 × 5 ml teaspoonfuls should be taken at night. Syrup: 10–20 ml should be taken as required.

Contraindications

Undiagnosed acute or persistent abdominal symptoms. Intestinal obstruction

Side effects
Excessive use may lead to potassium deficiency and atonic non-functioning colon on prolonged usage and colonic ulceration. Overdosage leads to griping and diarrhoea.

Special features
Diabetic patients should take the tablets as these have a low sugar content.

Danthron, BP (dihydroxyanthraquinone)
Dihydroxyanthraquinone is marketed combined with dioctyl sodium sulphosuccinate. This is not recommended, since DSS is considered hepatotoxic. It is also available with poloxamer 200 mg as Dorbanex (Riker), and one-to-two capsules (5–10 ml) at bedtime may be used for constipation or prior to surgery.

Hydrophilic bulking agents. These may be considered under the following classifications: (a) dietary fibre, (b) bran fibre and bran cereals, and (c) pharmaceutical hydrophilic preparations.

Isphagula husk, BP
The pressure diseases of the large bowel (diverticular disease) may be treated by a daily regime of natural fibre. Daily Fybogel (Reckitt and Colman) therapy provides 7 g natural fibre (with a capacity to retain 40 times its own weight of water), thus preventing increased colonic segmentation and avoiding high intra-colonic pressures as well as reducing transit time. High-pressure straining episodes are also avoided, as evacuation of the faeces is easily achieved.

Presentation

Sachet	isphagula husk granules as a low-electrolyte product containing 0.4 mmol of sodium and 0.7 mmol of potassium per sachet.

Dose
One sachet should be taken morning and evening.

Contraindications
Intestinal obstruction, senile megacolon, and patients on a salt-restricted diet. Intestinal atony and faecal impaction.

Side effects
Abdominal distension and flatulence.

Special features
It is presented as an effervescent granule which gives an excellent dispersion in water to produce a bland drink; it should be made up as an orange or lime

drink and taken as soon as possible, since it gels rapidly; also available as a combination product with mebeverine hydrochloride (see below).

Bran (Fybranta; Norgine)

This presents bran 2 g mixed with calcium phosphate 100 mg in tablet form.

Dose

An oral dose of 6–12 tablets should be taken daily in divided doses. The tablets may be chewed or taken with liquid.

Contraindications

Intestinal obstruction and gluten enteropathy.

Special features

Fybranta is more expensive than ordinary bran; ordinary bran and other wholegrain products are available.

Spasmolytics. These are indicated for the reduction of the hypersegmentation and exaggerated intraluminal pressures, which are characteristic of the irritable bowel syndrome, for diverticulitis and for the relief of pain.

Mebeverine hydrochloride

This is an antispasmodic, but does not affect the normal gut motility. It does not act via the autonomic nervous system and is not prone to the side effects of the anticholinergic antispasmodics, such as dry mouth, blurred vision, urinary retention and constipation.

Presentation

Tablets 135 mg.

Dose

An oral dose of 135 mg should be taken three times a day, 20 minutes before meals.

Contraindications

Paralytic ileus and porphyria..

Side effects

None serious.

Special features

It is not prone to the side effects of the anticholinergic antispasmodics.

Enemata. These are mainly used for the evacuation of impacted faeces, clearance of faecal accumulations in midwifery and bowel clearance for endoscopy, radiology or surgery. Soap enemata, previously fashionable, are now considered unacceptable because of side effects including mucosal damage and systemic effects from the rapid depletion of body water, hyperkalaemia and haemoconcentration, while chemical stimulant enemas including glycerin and Micralax (Evans Medical Limited) are all considered of questionable value. More acceptable methods include large-volume washouts, oil-retention enemas, small-volume saline washouts, disposable hypertonic saline enemas and suppositories.

Fletchers' arachis oil retention enema (Pharmax)
This contains arachis oil, BP, 130 ml. It is especially useful to soften impacted or hard faeces if local anal lesions are present.

Phosphates enema, BP
This is available in two formulas. Formula A: 100 ml sodium acid phosphate 16% w/v and sodium phosphate 6% w/v in purified water. Formula B: 128 ml sodium acid phosphate 10% w/v and sodium phosphate 8% w/v, in purified water.

Presentation
Disposable pack single-dose enema of 128ml.

Dose
One, as required, should be administered at room temperature or after warming in warm water.

Contraindications
These are applicable to all enemas and include antepartum haemorrhage, premature labour, probable urinary-tract infection, unstable lie and also any increased absorptive capacity of the colon.

Side effects
Hypersensitivity.

Special features
None known.

Suppositories
These are only mildly stimulant and lubricating, but have modest success, e.g. glycerine suppositories.

Infusions

The content, indications and contraindications of simple intravenous infusions are shown in Table 10.4 Solutions are available for intravenous parenteral feeding, but these are rarely required in gynaecological practice and should be used after consultation with physicians specializing in metabolic problems. The addition of drugs to intravenous solutions may be hazardous and should preferably be undertaken by the clinical pharmacist.

Radiological contrast media

Echovist 200 (S.H.U.454)

This suspension of galactose monosaccharide microparticles in a 20% aqueous solution is used during hysterosalpingo-contrast-sonography to assess tubal patency.

Iodised oil viscous injection, BP 1963

This is a sterile iodine addition product of the ethyl esters of the fatty acids of poppyseed oil (38% w/v of combined iodine). Oil embolism has been associated with this preparation when used near a menstrual period or when the endometrium or cervix has been subject to recent trauma. Water-soluble preparations are therefore advisable and include the following.

Diaginol viscous (May and Baker)

This is a sterile solution of sodium acetrizoate 40% w/v, with the addition of dextran to increase the viscosity.

Special features

Some degree of pain is occasionally complained of, although it may be difficult to distinguish that due to instrumentation and that due to the medium. Some discomfort may be experienced when the medium enters the pelvic peritoneal cavity.

Urografin 370 (76%) (Schering Chemicals)

This intravenous injection contains meglumine diatrizoate (66% w/v) and sodium diatrizoate 10% w/v containing iodine 370 mg/ml. It is well suited for intravenous urography and hysterosalpingography.

Special features

Mild subjective symptoms, such as sensation of heat or nausea, which rapidly disappear after slowing down the injection, have been noted.

Conray 420 (May and Baker)

This is indicated for intravenous urography. It contains sodium iothalamate 70% w/v containing 420 mg iodine in combined form per ml.

Side effects

Nausea, vomiting, dizziness and urticaria have been reported.

Table 10.4 Infusions

Solution	Indication	Electrolytes (mmol/l)	Contraindications/ side effects
(A) Sodium chloride 0.9% w/v	Post-operative fluid replacement	Na^+(150), Cl^- (150)	It should not be administered rapidly or for prolonged periods, since sudden cardiac arrest or circulatory overloading may occur. Venous thrombosis may occur
(B) Dextrose 4% w/v with sodium chloride 0.18% w/v	Post-operative fluid replacement	Na^+(30), Cl^-(30)	It should not be administered rapidy or for prolonged periods, since sudden cardiac arrest or circulatory overloading may occur. Venous thrombosis may occur. Diabetes is a contraindication. Dextrose solutions may be hazardous in patients with impaired hepatic or renal function. Rapid administration of large volumes may cause water intoxication. Infusion over a long period may cause dehydration
(C) Hartmann's solution (compound sodium lactate)	Post-operative fluid replacement	Na^+(131) K^+(5) Ca^{2+}(2) Cl^-(111) HCO^-_3 (29)	This should not be administered to patients with severe liver damage who would be unable to convert lactate to bicarbonate. It should be used with caution in patients with cardiac failure, hypertension, impaired renal function, pulmonary oedema and toxaemia of pregnancy. Venous thrombosis may occur

Table 10.4 Continued

Solution	Indication (mmol/l)	Electrolytes (mmol/l)	Contraindications/ side effects
(D) Dextrose 5%, 10%	For correction of ketosis	—	As for (B) above
(E) Dextran 40, 70	For prophylaxis of deep-vein thrombosis and improvement of peripheral perfusion	—	Group and cross-matching of blood should be undertaken *before* infusion. Allergy and hypersensitivity occasionally occurs; pyrexia, urticaria; tachycardia and dyspnoea may arise. Anaphylaxis has been reported
Dextran 70	For fluid replacement; it acts as a plasma expander	—	
Dextran 110	For fluid replacement; it acts as a plasma expander	—	
(F) Sodium bicarbonate 8.4%	For correction of acidosis, e.g. cardiac arrest	Na^+ (150) HCO_3 (150)	The administration of sodium bicarbonate may induce pulmonary oedema in patients receiving cardiopulmonary resuscitation

Hypersensitivity may occur with all contrast media. Minor symptoms such as itchy skin, sneezing, violent yawns, tickling of the throat, hoarseness or attacks of coughing may be early signs of a severe reaction and merit careful attention. Major symptoms should be treated with steroids, plasma substitutes and oxygen.

Non-specific local agents

Baths (salt baths)

This is a traditional form of therapy following pelvic surgery, especially if complicated by vault haematomas. Based on a bath size of 120 litres average, sodium chloride 4.2 kg would be required to give a 3.5% w/v concentration equivalent to that of the salt concentration in sea water. Salt baths rarely have this concentration of salt and this traditional therapy is therefore of questionable value.

Brilliant green and crystal violet paint, BP (Bonney's blue paint)

Formulation

Crystal violet and brilliant green in equal parts to make a 1% solution in 50% alcohol. This may be used as a cleansing agent for vaginal preparation prior to abdominal hysterectomy or vaginal surgery.

Glycerol, BP, Eur.P, USP (glycerin)

This hygroscopic preparation is used for resolving vault haematomas. It absorbs water and is dehydrating but irritating to exposed tissue. Concentrated solutions are slowly bactericidal.

Indigo carmine, BP (indigotindisulfonate, sodium USP)

Presentation

Injection
  Indigotindisulfonate
  Indigo carmine

Dose

An intramuscular injection of 50–100 mg may be given or 40–80 mg may be given by intravenous injection.

Contraindications

None known.

Indications

It is advised as a renal function test at cystoscopy, or used for assistance in the diagnosis of a vesicovaginal fistula or ruptured membranes.

Side effects

Nausea, vomiting, hypertension, bradycardia and skin reactions.

Special features

It may be given direct into the bladder to help in the diagnosis of vesicovaginal fistula.

Methylene blue injection, USP

Presentation

Injection 100 mg/10 ml.

Dose

A dose of 0.1–0.2 ml/kg body weight should be given by slow intravenous injection.

Contraindications

None known.

Indications
It is used as a renal function test at cystoscopy, or is used to assist in the diagnosis of vesicovaginal fistula or ruptured membranes.

Side effects
Nausea, abdominal and pre-cordial pain, dizziness, headache, profuse sweating, mental confusion, and the formation of methaemoglobin.

Special features
It should be given slowly by intravenous injection to prevent local high concentrations of the compound producing methaemoglobinaemia (low concentrations, however, convert methaemoglobin to haemoglobin). It may be given direct into the bladder.

Phenazopyridine hydrochloride USP (Pyridium; Warner)

Presentation
Tablets 100 mg.

Dose
An oral dose of two tablets should be taken three times a day before meals.

Contraindications
Patients with glomerular nephritis, uraemia, or severe hepatitis.

Indications
It has been used to help in the diagnosis of ruptured membranes. It is also advised as a urinary-tract analgesic for the relief of pain and dysuria in common urogenital infections.

Side effects
Large doses lead to methaemoglobinaemia.

Special features
After taking Pyridium, the urine becomes orange to red in colour for 2–3 days. Pyridium may be used concurrently with any sulphonamide, antibiotic or urinary antiseptic.

Schiller's iodine
Its use has been advocated prior to cone biopsy to outline any abnormal epithelium. Normal cervical epithelium stains brown because of its glycogen content, but in dysplasia and carcinoma the abnormal epithelium is deficient in glycogen and fails to stain. However, several benign conditions do not take up the stain for the same reason.

Further reading

Berggyist, D. *et al.* (1992). Prevention of venous thromboembolism after surgery: a review of enoxaparin. *British Journal of Surgery,* **79**, 495–498.

Degenhard, F.F. *et al.* (1993). Vaginal hysterosalpingo-contrast-sonography. *Bruus Bulletin*, November.

Drug and Therapeutics Bulletin (1992). **30**(30) How to anticoagulate.

Gruber, U.F. *et al.* (1980). Incidences of fatal postoperative pulmonary embolism after prophylaxis with dextran 70 and low dose heparin: an international multicentre study. *British Medical Journal,* **i**, 69–72.

Lowe, G.D.O. *et al.* (1992). Risk of and prophylaxis for venous thromboembolism in hospital patients. *British Medical Journal,* **305,** 567–574.

Prandon. P., Lensing, A.W.A., Buller, H.R. *et al.* (1992). Comparison of subcutaneous low molecular weight heparin with intravenous standard heparin in proximal deep vein thrombosis. *Lancet,* 339, 441–445.

Oral Anticooagulants; British National Formulary No 27 (March 1994) pp 99

The UK approach as regards these topics differs considerably from procedures in the United States and are considered separately in Appendix I and II..

Appendix I

Abortion, Fertility Control, Hirsutism and Lactation Suppression

Introduction

There are many who would encourage practitioners to contribute to a reduction of population by advising on methods of fertility control. Globally, a population growth rate of 1.7% per annum approximates at present, giving a yearly natural increase of 72 millions. Breast feeding provides partial contraception, but more sophisticated means of family planning are available and should reduce the need for termination of pregnancy, which however in some communities, appears to be the elected method of choice.

Abortion

Abortion has many subdivisions.

Threatened and recurrent abortions

Progestogens have been used in the management of cases of threatened and recurrent abortions, but there is no evidence from controlled trials that they are of specific benefit and the good results frequently obtained are probably due to overall psychological support. If patients have previously received them with a successful outcome and request further therapy, then only those drugs, e.g. hydroxyprogesterone hexanoate, which have no masculinizing effects on any female fetus, may be used. Where systemic lupus erythematosis is diagnosed as causing recurrent miscarriages, heparin therapy 5000 s.c. twice daily from conception to 14 weeks is advocated.

Progesterone BP, Eur.P, USP (see p. 152)

Progestogens are also used as contraceptives (see p. 152), for post-partum depression and for the suppression of lactation (see p. 158). Other indications include dysfunctional uterine bleeding (see p. 72), dysmenorrhoea (see p. 61) and endometriosis (see p. 64), and carcinoma of the corpus uteri (see p. 163).

Hydroxyprogesterone hexanoate, BP (hydroxyprogesterone caproate, USP)

Presentation

Injection 250 mg, 500 mg

Dose

Habitual abortion:	250–500 mg should be given weekly by intramuscular injection during the first half of the pregnancy.
Threatened abortion:	500 mg should be given daily by intramuscular injection until the bleeding stops. Then 250–500 mg should be given intramuscularly in three doses every 3 days, and weekly throughout the first half of pregnancy.

Contraindications

A history of gestational herpes.

Indications

Progestogen therapy may have a place in a few problem cases where there is habitual abortion of normal fetuses and where there has been a thorough investigation in a specialized unit.

Side effects

Local reactions at the injection site may occur.

Special features

None.

Other progestogens used in the management of habitual abortion include **allyloestrenol**, **dydrogesterone** (see p. 61) and pure progesterone (see p. 76).

Allyloestrenol

Presentation

Tablets 5 mg.

Dose

An oral dose of 5–10 mg daily for at least 16 weeks.

Contraindications
Patients with thrombotic disease or mammary carcinoma.

Side effects
A decreased glucose tolerance may occur in diabetic patients.

Special features
Allyloestrenol is used where failure of nidation is thought to be due to lack of progesterone. The dose is 10–20 mg daily, from the 16th to the 26th day of each cycle until conception is achieved, and then 10 mg daily for at least 16 weeks.

First trimester abortions

After appropriate counselling, patients may be accepted for termination of pregnancy under the UK Abortion Act 1967 (amended 1991). With the availability of liberal contraceptive methods, minimal abortions should be indicated, but 170,000 abortions are still undertaken in the UK per annum. Fortunately, there are now almost no septic abortions which were previously associated with illegal abortions, which previously required concentrated antibiotic coverage and intensive therapy (see p. 33).

Surgical termination of pregnancy

Early abortions may be performed as day-case procedures using minimal analgesia such as diazepam and pethidine mixtures (Demerol, USP) which are most suitable. In young primigravidae, general anaesthesia is preferable after cervical ripening, using prostaglandin pessaries.

Diazepam 10 mg should be given intravenously and followed after 5 minutes by pethidine hydrochloride 100 mg and promethazine hydrochloride 50 mg. The diazepam is used to allay apprehension and the pethidine for analgesic effects. Promethazine is also an antihistamine anti-emetic with relaxing properties. The combination of drugs provides excellent analgesia for minor gynaecological procedures.

Gemeprost

This prostaglandin is specifically indicated pre-operatively for softening and dilatation of the cervix to facilitate transcervical operative procedures in the first trimester when inserted into the posterior fornix 3 hours prior to surgery. For second trimester terminations, 1 mg is used every 3 hours to a maximum 5 times repeating the process after 24 hours if necessary.

Presentation
Pessaries 1 mg.

Dose
1 mg 3 hours prior to surgery.

Contraindications
Obstructive airways disease, cardiovascular insufficiency, raised intra-ocular pressure.

Side effects
Vaginal bleeding, uterine pain, nausea, vomiting or diarrhoea; headache, muscle weakness, dizziness, flushing, chills, backache, dyspnoea, chest pain, palpitations, mild pyrexia; rarely uterine rupture.

Special features
Especially indicated for the very young primigravida with a tight cervical os.

Diazepam, BP, USP
This is a mild tranquillizer and a nocturnal sedative; it has muscle-relaxant properties.

Presentation

Syrup	2 mg/5 ml
Tablets	2 mg, 5 mg, 10 mg
Capsules	2 mg, 5 mg
Ampoules	5 mg/ml

Dose
Intravenous injections 10 mg, in combination with pethidine and promethazine; it is also given orally, 2 or 5mg one to three times a day, and 5 mg up to 50 mg (maximum) may be given by injection.

Contraindications
Nil specific.

Indications
To allay apprehension, in combination with analgesics and anti-emetic drugs for minor gynaecological surgery.

Side effects
Diazepam may cause thrombophlebitis when given by intravenous injection, but it is available in an oil–water emulsion to greatly reduce the incidence of this problem. It should be used with care when other central nervous system depressants are given, as the side effects may be synergistic.

Promethazine hydrochloride, BP, Eur.P, USP

This is a long-acting phenothiazine derivative and has anti-emetic, antihistaminic and relaxing properties.

Presentation

Ampoules	25 mg/ml, 1 ml, 2 ml
Tablets	10 mg, 25 mg
Syrup	5 mg/5 ml

Dose

Intravenous injection of 50 mg, in combination with pethidine for minor gynaecological surgery. It may also be used as a sedative, 25–50 mg orally or by injection at night.

Contraindications

Patients with a history of convulsions, intracranial trauma or severe hypotension should not receive promethazine hydrochloride.

Indications

To enhance the analgesic effect of pethidine (meperidine) hydrochloride and act as an anti-emetic sedative for minor gynaecological surgery. It may also be used as a sedative.

Side effects

The patient should not drive or take alcohol. It will enhance the action of any sedative, hypnotic or other central nervous system sedative.

Special features

It is also used as an anti-emetic in early pregnancy and in labour to enhance the effect of pethidine (meperidine) hydrochloride.

Pethidine hydrochloride, BP, USP, Eur.P (meperidine hydrochloride, USP; Demerol, USP)

This is a narcotic analgesic and is subject to the UK Misuse of Drugs Act 1971. It has analgesic and antispasmodic properties, is relatively short acting and has little soporific effect.

Presentation

Tablets	50 mg
Injection	50 mg/ml, 100 mg/2 ml

Dose

Intravenous injection of 100 mg for minor gynaecological procedures

Contraindications

Patients receiving monoamine oxidase inhibitors or within 2 weeks of their withdrawal, respiratory depression or obstructive airways disease. It should be used with caution in patients with severe hepatic impairment, biliary-tract disorders, hypothyroidism, adrenocortical insufficiency, supraventricular tachycardia or convulsive disorders.

Side effects

Mild euphoria, dizziness, nausea and vomiting, hypotension and respiratory depression.

Special features

Potentiates other central nervous system depressants and phenothiazines with possible severe hypotension.

Medical termination of pregnancy

Mifepristone

During pregnancy, circulating progesterone inhibits uterine contractions and the use of a progesterone antagonist — mifepristone — induces abortions in 60–85% of women when used alone and 94–98% of women if coupled with a vaginal pessary of gemeprost 36–48 hours later. The contractility of the uterus is much greater than with either compound alone.

Mifepristone is a synthetic steroid molecule with a chemical structure similar to that of progesterone — it is an antiprogesterone which inhibits the effects of progesterone by blocking its activity at the intracellular receptor.

Presentation

Tablets 200 mg.

Dose

A single oral dose of 600 mg is given in the presence of a doctor or nurse. (After 36–48 hours, if the abortion is incomplete, a vaginal pessary of gemeprost 1 mg is inserted; see p. 136.) The patient should be observed for 6 hours and reviewed after 12 days.

Contraindications

Heavy smokers, women over 35 years and women with cardiovascular disease. Mifepristone blocks the effects of glucocorticoids and should not be used in women with chronic adrenal failure or those on long-term corticosteroid therapy. It is contraindicated in women with haemorrhagic disorders or those on anticoagulant therapy and is not effective in terminating ectopic pregnancies.

Side effects
It is not indicated in patients with asthma or chronic obstructive airways disease, or women with renal or hepatic failure.

Special features
It is restricted to use where the pregnancy is less than 63 days from the last menstrual period.

Second trimester abortions

In the UK, the most common procedure is to employ prostaglandin $E_2\alpha$ vaginally. The intra-amniotic or extra-amniotic route is occasionally used, coupled with oxytocin infusion to whose effects the uterus may have been sensitized by the prostaglandin. Alternative intra-amniotic hypertonic solutions previously used include hypertonic saline, urea, dextrose or mannitol, but none is without risk. Hypertonic saline with a small chance of intravenous leakage may cause maternal damage to the brain; urea, saline and glucose have been associated with consumption coagulopathy and haemorrhage.

For evacuation of the uterus with missed abortion or hydatidiform mole, intravenous infusion of prostaglandin E_2 is the treatment of choice for both these conditions. If haemorrhage should occur, intravenous ergometrine with oxytocin infusions is indicated.

Prostaglandins. These are long-chain unsaturated fatty acids containing a 5-carbon ring along their length and are derivatives of a hypothetical molecule 'prostanoic acid'. They are found in most tissues and in especially high concentration in seminal fluid from the seminal vesicles. There are four major groups of naturally occurring prostaglandins — E, F, A and B; the prostaglandins E_2 and $F_2\alpha$ are of most importance in gynaecology.

Dinoprostone (prostaglandin E_2)
This is used in the form of gels or vaginal pessaries for softening the cervix before termination of pregnancy; in intra- or extra-amniotic infusion for intra-uterine fetal death; and as an intravenous infusion for hydatidiform mole, missed abortion or intra-uterine death. Vaginal prostaglandin E_2 may be used to facilitate surgical evacuation of the uterus.

Presentation

Vaginal gel	400 µg/ml, 800 µg/ml in disposable syringes (Total doses 1mg, 2mg in 2.5ml syringes)
Cervical gel	200 µg/ml in disposable syringes (Total dose = 500 µg in 2.5ml)

Vaginal tablets	3 mg
Tablets (oral)	500 µg
Vaginal tablets	3 mg
Intravenous solution	1 mg/ml, 0.75 ml for intravenous infusion
Extra-amniotic solution	10 mg/ml, 0.5 ml for extra-amniotic infusion

Dose

Pre-operative cervical ripening. A tablet is applied to the posterior vaginal fornix and repeated if required in 6–8 hours (2 × 3 mg maximum dose).

Second trimester termination of pregnancy. Prostaglandin E_2, 10 mg, by intra-amniotic injection, repeated if necessary in 12–24 hours. A 5 mg ampoule dissolved in 50 ml of the manufacturer's diluent to give a solution of 100 µg/ml may be used for extra-amniotic infusion. 1 ml is instilled into the extra-amniotic space using a No. 12 French gauge (o.d. 4 mm) Foley catheter with the balloon distended with 15–20 ml sterile water and depending on the uterine response, followed with 1–2 ml of prostaglandin solution every 2 hours.

Evacuation of hydatidiform mole, missed abortion or intra-uteruine death. Prostaglandin E_2, a 5 µg/ml solution in 0.9% saline or 5% dextrose, is infused at 2.5 µg per minute for 30 minutes and then maintained or increased to 5 µg per minute according to response and side effects. The dose is maintained for at least 4 hours before increasing further, if necessary, to produce or enhance uterine contractions.

Contraindications

Previous caesarean section or other major uterine surgery. Raised ocular pressure or glaucoma.

Side effects

These include uterine hypertonia; nausea, vomiting and diarrhoea; headache and peripheral flushing occasionally occur.

Special features

Prostaglandins sensitize the uterus to oxytocin and oxytocin may be used in cautious doses to supplement or continue the effects of prostaglandins. The tablets are easy to use; the gels allow flexibility of dose and provide more rapid absorption.

Dinoprost (prostaglandin F_2)

Presentation

Ampoules	5 mg/ml, 4 ml, 8 ml
Intra-amniotic use	5 mg (as trometamol salt)/ml
Intravenous use	1.5 ml, 5 ml

Dose
Second trimester termination of pregnancy. Intra-amniotic use: 40 mg. Extra-amniotic use: 375 μg/ml via a Foley catheter, starting with 1 ml and adding 1–2 ml every 2 hours depending on uterine response; a similar schedule may also be used in cases of intra-uterine fetal death.

Contraindications
Raised intra-ocular pressure of glaucoma. Asthmatics: prostaglandin $F_2\alpha$ in constrast to prostaglandin E_2 has a mild bronchoconstrictor effect.

Side effects
As for prostaglandin E_2. With intravenous use, local tissue irritation and erythema may occur. A transient pyrexia and elevated white blood cell count are not uncommon, but require no specific management and resolve spontaneously.

Special features
This is indicated for hospital use only and is rarely used.

Hypertonic solutions. These include saline, urea, dextrose or mannitol. Dextrose hypertonic solutions have been associated with maternal deaths and are not to be recommended. They have been rarely used since the advent of prostaglandins.

Hypertonic saline

Presentation
18% Hypertonic saline (27 g sodium chloride).

Dose
Amniotic fluid 100–200 ml is withdrawn with a 50 ml syringe and 18% saline solution (100–200 ml maximum) injected slowly into the uterine cavity.

Contraindications
High-risk patients include women with sickle-cell disease, anaemia or cardiac or cardiovascular disorders.

Side effects
Intravascular or intraperitoneal injection will produce lower abdominal pain and a feeling of faintness or flushing, tingling or burning of the face, upper limbs or mouth. Haemorrhage due to consumption coagulopathy may occur and maternal deaths have been reported, mainly due to faulty technique.

Special features
The saline may be supplemented with an intravenous infusion of Syntocinon in 5% dextrose (100–200 units) with strict monitoring of fluid balance. Intra-

amniotic injections of antibiotics, such as benzylpenicillin 600 mg and streptomycin 500 mg, may be added to the injected solution.

Mannitol, BP, USP

Presentation
25% Mannitol injection, USP.

Dose
100–200 ml of amniotic fluid is removed and replaced with 200 ml of 25% mannitol.

Contraindications
Mannitol is not recommended where the fetus is past 16 weeks. After 16 weeks' gestation, the fetus may be aborted alive.

Side effects
Headache, nausea and vomiting may occur.

Special features
Nil specific.

Urea, BP, USP

Presentation
Hypertonic solution 40 g vial.

Dose
The amniotic fluid is replaced with hypertonic urea solution 200 ml (80 g in 200 ml 5% dextrose).

Contraindications
Marked impairment of hepatic or renal function, since it may confuse monitoring of liver and renal function

Side effects
Intravenous leakage may cause headache, nausea, vomiting, confusion and hypotension.

Special features
Prostaglandin E_2, 2.5–10 mg, may be injected intra-amniotically when the urea solution has been administered. The urea may also be supplemented by an intravenous oxytocin infusion, 100–176 U/litre, with strict monitoring of fluid balance.

Oxytocics. These may be used to supplement prostaglandin or hypertonic solutions given by injection or intravenous infusion in the management of haemorrhage following termination of pregnancy or delivery.

Oxytocin injection, BP, Eur.P, USP

Presentation

Ampoules	2 units in 2 ml
	5 units in 1 ml
	10 units in 1 ml
	50 units in 5 ml

Dose

For supplementation of prostaglandin/hypertonic	Oxytocin 5% in dextrose is given by titration to a maximum of 176 units/litre and maintained for 10–12 solutions.hours.
For management of post-partum haemorrhage	Oxytocin 50U/litre in 5% dextrose, 500 ml by titration at 25 Mu per minute (5 drops per minute with a 20 drops per minute infusion set) and increased to 50 Mu per minute(10 drops per minute) until the uterus contracts. The infusion should be maintained at this rate for 1 hour.

Side effects

A rapid intravenous injection of 5 units of oxytocin in concentrated solution can cause a transient hypotensive episode with tachycardia and an increase in pulmonary artery pressure. Water intoxication can occur, since oxytocin is an antidiuretic.

Ergometrine maleate, BP, Eur.P

This uterotonic drug is used in the management of spontaneous and legal abortion and in the management of post-partum haemorrhage due to uterine atony. It requires a hyperoestrogen situation to work effectively and is of no value in the management of non-obstetric haemorrhage.

Presentation

Injection 0.5 mg/ml.

Dose

An intravenous dose of 125–250 μg may be given to prevent or assist in arresting haemorrhage in relation to abortion. The dose may be repeated once in 10 minutes or 500μg given i.m.

Contraindications

Ergometrine maleate is best avoided in patients with heart disease or hypertension. It is contraindicated in patients with Raynaud's disease or other vasospastic disorders.

Side effects
Peripheral vasoconstriction and hypertension, nausea and vomiting. Rare cases of Raynaud's phenomenon, post-partum eclampsia and post-partum haemolytic uraemic syndrome have been reported.

Special features
A methyl derivative of ergometrine maleate (methylergonovine; dose 0.2 mg by intramuscular or intravenous injection) is available in the United States. Ergometrine maleate is also available in combination with oxytocin as Syntometrine (Sandoz).

Control of fertility

Advice relating to fertility control should be offered to all patients in the reproductive years. This may be in general practice at any consultation, if appropriate, and even in the pre-pregnancy clinic its use can be discussed. Fertility control should also be discussed during counselling for termination of pregnancy, which should be a non-recurring clinical condition.

There are many monographs available on fertility control including that by Hawkins and Elder (1979). A directory of contraceptives is published (Carne *et al.*, 1979) which lists the availability of contraceptives on a worldwide coverage.

This section relates specifically to oral contraceptives and long acting contraceptives including subdermal implants. Intra-uterine devices, spermicidal creams and pessaries are also mentioned.

Steroid contraceptives

Steroid contraceptives may contain either a pure progestogen or, more normally, an oestrogen and progestogen combined. The oestrogens used include ethinyloestradiol and its 3-methyl ether, mestranol. The progestogens are related to the parent compounds 19-nortestosterone and 17-α-hydroxyprogesterone, although at present all preparations available in the UK rely on 19-nortestosterone derivatives.

The combined preparation acts by suppression of ovulation (the oestrogens suppress the release of gonadotrophin-releasing hormone so that the pituitary production of follicle-stimulating hormone is reduced) and it also acts on the endometrium and cervical mucus. Combination type oral contraceptives decrease the risk of endometrial and ovarian cancer but increase the risk of liver cancer.

The progestogens produce a pseudodecidual reaction that prevents implantation and they also act on cervical mucus making it impenetrable to sperm. The 19-norsteroid, norethisterone, may also inhibit ovulation or disturb ovarian steroidogenesis. Most progestogens have some oestrogenic action, but levonorgestrel is devoid of any oestrogen activity.

Oral therapy.

Presentation
Tablets of combined preparations with a maximum of 50 μg of oestrogen or single progestogen tablets only (with or without placebo). See Tables A.1 to A.3.

Dose
Combined preparations. 21 tablets: 1 tablet daily should be taken from day 1, 2, 3 or 4 of the menstrual cycle. 28 tablets: 1 tablet daily should be taken from day 5 of the menstrual cycle and 7 placebo tablets taken daily throughout the menstrual cycle. These tablets are especially useful for post-partum patients.

Contraindications
Considerable debate continues as to whether it is acceptable to prescribe the oral contraceptive to women over 34 years of age who have had one or more of the other predisposing risk factors for ischaemic heart disease and thromboembolism, i.e. diabetes, obesity, heavy smoking, treated hypertension or type II hyperlipidaemia. The US Food and Drug Administration has recommended that women aged 40 years and over should not take oral contraceptives; the British Committee on Safety of Medicines is keeping the situation under review and has issued the following statements:

> The risk of arterial thrombosis associated with combined oral contraceptive increases with age and this risk is aggravated by cigarette smoking. The use of combined oral contraceptives by women in the older age group, especially those who are cigarette smokers, should therefore be discouraged and alternative methods advised.

Many patients may elect a definitive method of contraception, i.e. sterilization, but others prefer to continue on low-dose oral contraceptives for many years, even up to, and throughout, the menopause. The clinician should advise the patient of potential hazards and monitor her weight and blood pressure regularly, with a routine 6-monthly or yearly gynaecological assessment, including cervical smear.

It may be acceptable for the woman to continue taking the oral contraceptive until she is post-menopausal when she may elect hormone replacement therapy (see Chapter 7).

Table A.1 Steroid contraceptive tablets with 50 µg of oestrogen

Proprietary name (UK drugs)	Oestrogen (µg) (Ethinyloestradiol/Mestranol)	Progestogen (mg)	
Norinyl 1	50	Norethisterone	1.0
Ortho-Novin 1/50	50	Norethisterone	1.0
Ovran	50	Levonorgestrel	0.25

Table A.2 Steroid contraceptives with less than 50 µg of oestrogen

Proprietary name (UK drugs)	Oestrogen (µg) (ethinyloestradiol)	Progestogen (mg)	
Brevinor	35	Norethisterone	0.5
Cilest	35	Norgestimate	0.25
Conova 30	30	Ethynodiol diacetate	2.0
Dianette	35	Cyproterone	2.0
Eugynon 30	30	Levonorgestrel	0.25
Femodene	30	Gestodene	0.075
Loestrin 20	20	Norethisterone acetate	1.0
Loestrin 30	30	Norethisterone acetate	1.5
Logynon	30, 40	Levonorgestrel	0.05, 0.075, 0.125
Logynon ED	30, 40	Levonorgestrel	0.05, 0.075, 0.125
Marvelon	30	Desogestrel	0.15
Mercilon	20	Desogestrel	0.15
Microgynon-30	30	Levonorgestrel	0.15
Minulet	30	Gestodene	0.075
Neocon	35	Norethisterone	1.0
Norimin	35	Norethisterone	1.0
Ovran 30	30	Levonorgestrel	0.25
Ovran	50	Levonorgestrel	0.25
Ovranette	30	Levonorgestrel	0.15
Ovysmen	35	Norethisterone	0.5
Trinovum	35	Norethisterone	0.5, 0.75,1.0
Trinordiol	30, 40	Levonorgestrel	0.05, 0.075, 0.125
Triadene	30, 40	Gestodene	0.05, 0.07, 0.100
Tri-minulet	30, 40	Gestodene	0.05, 0.07, 0.100

Many alternative forms are available in different countries and the UK formulations are listed as examples. Dianette (Schering) is best reserved for patients being treated for androgen dependent skin conditions (see p. 156).

Table A.3 Progestogen-only steroid contraceptive tablets

Proprietary name (UK drugs)	Progestogen (mg)	
Femulen	Ethynodiol diacetate	0.5
Micronor	Norethisterone	0.35
Microval	Levonorgestrel	0.03
Neogest	DL-Norgestrel	0.075
Noriday	Norethisterone	0.35
Norgeston	Levonorgestrel	0.03

Table A.4 Estimates of risk of death from pulmonary embolism or cerebral thrombosis in users and non-users of oral contraceptives compared with risk of death from certain other causes

Risk factor	Age in years	
	20–34	35–44
Estimated annual death-rate from pulmonary or cerebral thromboembolism per 100,000 healthy, married non-pregnant women:		
Users of oral contraceptives	1.5	3.9
Non-users of oral contraceptives	0.2	0.2
Annual death rate* per 100,000 total female population from:		
Cancer	13.7	70.1
Motor accidents	4.9	3.9
All causes	60.1	170.5
Annual death rate* per 100,000 maternities from:		
Complications of pregnancy	7.5	13.8
Abortion	5.6	10.4
Complications of delivery	7.1	26.5
Complications of the puerperium:		
Phlebitis, thrombosis and embolism	1.3	2.3
Other complications	1.3	4.6
All risks of pregnancy, delivery and puerperium	22.8	57.6

*From the Registrar General's *Statistical Reviews of England and Wales* for 1966

Table A.5 The effects of drugs on oestrogen-progestogen oral contraceptives

Interacting drug	Effect of interaction
Analgesics:	
Amidopyrine	Breakthrough bleeding
Anticonvulsants:	
Methylphenobarbitone Phenobarbitone Phenytoin Primidone	Breakthrough bleeding, Contraceptive failure
Antimigraine:	
Dihydroergotamine	Contraceptive failure
Antituberculous and anti-infective agents:	
Ampicillin	Contraceptive failure
Chloramphenicol	Breakthrough bleeding, contraceptive failure
Nitrofurantoin	Breakthrough bleeding
Phenoxymethylpenicillin	
Rifampicin	Breakthrough bleeding, contraceptive failure
Sulphamethoxypyridazine	Contraceptive failure
Tranquillizers:	
Meprobamate	Contraceptive failure

Side effects

Reported side effects of combined oestrogen–progestogen preparations include the following:

1. Metabolic changes: thyroxine binding globulin, protein-bound iodine, transferrin, serum iron, triglycerol, and cholesterol and lipoprotein levels are all elevated.
2. Nausea.
3. Breast tenderness.
4. Amenorrhoea.
5. Oligomenorrhoea.

Table A.6 The effects of oral contraceptives on other drugs

Interacting drug	Effect of interaction
Anti-asthmatic agents	No interaction, but asthmatic condition is sometimes exacerbated
Anticoagulants: Dicoumarol	Anticoagulant effect reduced
Anticonvulsants	Changes in the control of epilepsy can occur
Antidepressants: Imipramine	Antidepressant effects reduced: possible development of toxic effects
Antihypertensives: Guanethidine	Contraception-induced hypertension inadequately controlled
Hypoglycaemic agents: Insulin	Control of diabetes sometimes reduced due to the hyperglycaemic effects of oral contraceptives

6. Weight gain.
7. Hypertension — both components of the Pill may be responsible for this disturbance. The renin–angiotensin system is thought to be involved and renin substrate (angiotensinogen) levels are elevated by increasing doses of oestrogen. Hence, low oestrogen and non-oestrogenic progestogens (norgestrel) should be prescribed.
8. Liver damage.
9. Depression.
10. Fluid retention.
11. Carbohydrate metabolism: an increase in blood sugar and impaired glucose tolerance test have been demonstrated in some women, especially those with a diabetic family history.
12. Thrombotic episodes (Table A.4). — The Committee on Safety of Medicines recommended in 1969 that the dose of oestrogens in oral contraceptives should not exceed 50 μg to reduce thrombotic hazards. Research continues to assess whether any particular progestogen–oestrogen combination carries a larger risk of thrombosis.
13. Vertebral artery occlusion.
14. Endometrial carcinoma — sequential agents have been suggested as possible aetiological agents.
15. Hepatic vein occlusion.
16. Gallstones.
17. Myocardial infarction.

18. Hepatic neoplasia — these have been described as benign hepatomas, haematomas and focal nodular hyperplasia. They all have prominent vasculature and may present with massive bleeding into the peritoneal cavity.
19. Breast neoplasia — the Committee on Safety of Medicines has advised the withdrawal of oral contraceptives containing megestrol acetate because of the association with the development of tumours in the breasts of beagle bitches. Several studies have shown no association between the Pill and breast cancer in women and suggest that when taken for more than 2 years, the Pill decreases the risk of developing benign breast tumours.
20. Drug interactions with oral contraceptives (Tables A.5 and A.6) — breakthrough bleeding or spotting may indicate that other drugs may be interacting with the oral contraceptive affecting absorption or metabolism.
21. Galactorrhoea — this may indicate an underlying pituitary tumour and investigations should be considered, including serum prolactin levels.

Special features

1. Hyperplastic features in the cervix occur, leading to an increased vaginal discharge. Cytological changes may, however, occur secondarily to increased sexual activity, possibly with trichomonal infection. Yearly cervical cytology is indicated.
2. Varicose veins are *not* a contraindication to oral contraceptives. Provided that previous thrombotic disease is excluded and attention is paid to other factors such as obesity or possible elective surgery in the future, and patients are followed up regularly, then low-dose oestrogens do not seem to increase the risk of serious complications in a patient with superficial varicose veins.
3. Patients taking oral contraceptives during the months prior to surgery have an increased incidence of post-operative deep-vein thrombosis. This issue of discontinuing the oral contraceptive before surgery is one of weighing up risks; those of an unwanted pregnancy (if less reliable methods of contraception fail) should be balanced against the potential hazard of a thrombosis. Prophylactic techniques against deep-vein thrombosis are now available, including antithrombotic stockings or subcuticular heparin (5000 units twice daily) (see p. 115). The oral contraceptive should not be discontinued prior to minor surgery.
4. While the relative efficacy and safety of the oral contraceptive is accepted, the routine follow-up assessment should be mandatory and should include 6-monthly interview, blood pressure and weight check, and examination of the breasts and pelvis, including cervical smear and urine testing.

5. Cyproterone acetate with ethinyloestradiol contains an anti-androgen and is used as an oral contraceptive for women who are being treated for androgen-dependent skin conditions including acne and hirsutism. Hirsutism is a common and distressing problem and due to the action of androgens on the skin either due to excessive production by the ovary or increased tissue sensitivity to these androgens. Anti-androgens are used to control excessive hair growth (see p. 156).

Progestogen-only preparations

These preparations are less efficient than the oestrogen–progestogen mixtures, but they serve a useful function in those patients for whom oestrogen is contraindicated or who are intolerant of the mixed Pill.

Medroxyprogesterone acetate, BP, USP

Presentation

Ampoules 150 mg/ml in 1 ml,

Dose

Should be given by intramuscular injection; 150 mg at the beginning of the menstrual cycle or early in the puerperium.

Contraindications

Thrombophlebitis, a history of pulmonary embolism or liver dysfunction, or any suspected malignancy of the breast or genital organs.

Indications

It is advised as a short-term antifertility agent when an oral contraceptive is contraindicated or considered inappropriate. It is specifically advised as a post-vasectomy contraceptive or to provide cover after immunization against rubella. Used for long-term contraception it should be repeated every 3 months.

Side effects

In normal menstruating women, additional precautions against pregnancy should be taken 14 days following the injection.

Norethisterone enanthate

Presentation

Injection	200 mg/ml
Oral tablets	ethynodiol diacetate 500 µg
	norethisterone 350 µg
	levonorgestrel 30 µg
	norgestrel 75 µg

Indication
Suitable for short-term contraception; 200 mg intramuscularly in first 5 days of the cycle or immediately post-partum; recommended where oestrogens are contraindicated or not tolerated.

Dose
One tablet should be taken daily every day throughout the year, commencing on day 1 of the cycle, and continued without interruption as required.

Contraindications
These include thrombotic or cerebrovascular disorders of hormonal-dependent carcinoma. Other relative contraindications include biliary cirrhosis, impaired hepatic excretory function, the Dubin–Johnson syndrome, the rotor syndrome, jaundice, severe liver disease, carcinoma of the breast and genital tract, a history of thromboembolism, nulliparous patients with poor ovarian function, incomplete growth in a young girl, sickle-cell anaemia, and deterioration of otosclerosis during previous pregnancies.

Side effects
The major disadvantage of progestogen preparations is frequent and irregular bleeding, and they are less efficient than combined oral contraceptives owing to a single effect on the cervical mucus (but in some women, ovulation may also be depressed). Disordered tubal function and an increased ectopic pregnancy rate may be related.

Special features
They cause fewer endocrine alterations and probably have fewer dangerous effects on venous thrombosis and carbohydrate tolerance than oestrogens.

Long-acting contraception

There are several long-acting immediately-reversible contraceptives available including:

1. Copper intra-uterine devices
2. Subdermal implants releasing nevonorgestrel; considerable research is in press regarding different subdermal implants (Mascarenha L. (1994); one example is 'Norplant' (Cassenne) is a subdermal (progesterone only) hormonal contraceptive which provides effective contraception for up to 5 years. It consists of six small capsules containing levonorgestrel, a synthetic progesterone. These are placed under the skin of the inner aspect of the upper arm using special inserters, under local anaesthesia. They have to be removed after 5 years, which also needs a small procedure performed under local anaesthesia.

Chemistry and pharmokinetics

The progesterone used in 'Norplant' is levonorgestrel which is a 21-carbon, synthetic derivative of testosterone. The serum levels of the hormone in the first week of use are 1–2 ng/ml and these levels rapidly decline in the ensuing weeks to a plateau, between 0.25 ng.ml and 0.4 ng/ml by 6 months.

The steroid hormone is placed in capsules made from medical grade elastomer consisting of a dimethyesiloxane/methylvinylsiloxane co-polymer.

Presentation

It is prescribed as a Norplant set. One pack contains six capsules each filled with 38 mg of levonorgestrel for use by a single woman and packaged in a sterile, sealed, plastic pouch.
Each capsule is about 34 mm long, 2.4 mm in diameter.

Mode of action

Primary contraceptive effects are mainly two: firstly it causes thickening of the cervical mucus rendering it impenetrable by spermatozoa. It also prevents ovulation in around 50% of menstrual cycles. The secondary contraceptive effect is by causing endometrial hyperplasia and decrease in the secretion of progesterone in the luteal phase of those cycles in which ovulation does occur.

Contraindications

Known or suspected pregnancy, sensitivity to levonorgestrel, undiagnosed vaginal bleeding, sex hormone dependent neoplasia, acute liver disease, past history of thrombo-embolic disease, hypertension, familial hypercholesterolemia, recent trophoblastic disease, migraine, etc. Drug interactions are similar to those of other hormonal contraceptive drugs.

Starting Norplant

Most preferably on day 1 of the menstrual cycle. If inserted on other days, care should be taken to rule out pregnancy and to provide appropriate contraception for that cycle (generally for the next 7 days). Post abortion, it should be inserted within 5 days. Post child birth, it should be inserted after the first 21 days taking appropriate additional precautions for the next 7 days.

Efficacy

The worldwide experience of Norplant has produced a failure rate of 0.2 per 100 woman-years of Norplant use for the first 2 years and 0.9, 0.5 and 1.1 per 100 woman-years for the subsequent 3 years. More recent data puts the first year failure of Norplant at 0.04. This compares favourably with other methods simply because there can be no "user" failure with Norplant, unlike most other methods. The efficacy of the older Norplant was slightly reduced in obese women, but the introduction of a newer device has eliminated that problem.

The continuation rate in the first year is 75–90% and that in the 5th year is 25–50%. The average duration of use is around 3½ years.

Adverse effects

Problems associated with the surgical procedure such as infection or expulsion are rare. A change in menstrual pattern is the most common finding. There is a loss of the usual cyclicity and there can be prolonged bleeding (usually in the first months), intermenstrual bleeding or spotting, periods of amenorrhoea and increase or decrease in the number of days of bleeding. There is, however, no increase in the average loss of blood over a period of one year, as compared to loss prior to Norplant use. Headaches, nervousness, dizziness, nausea, acne, change in appetite, hirsutism, loss of scalp hair, adnexal enlargement (ovarian cysts), hyperpigmentation over implantation site are the other side effects noted.

Special features

The contraceptive action of Norplant starts within 24 hours of insertion. The contraceptive effect is reversible almost immediately upon removal, with prompt return to usual fertility.

Emergency contraception

Combined oral contraceptives may be given for occasional emergency use after unprotected intercourse. Two tablets of levonorgestrel 250 µg and ethinyloestradiol 50 µg are taken within 72 hours and a further two tablets 12 hours later. The patient should be reviewed 3 weeks after therapy.

Presentation

Ethinyloestradiol	50 µg +
Levonorgestrel	250 µg

Spermicidal creams and pessaries

These are advised for patients using barrier methods of contraception or for perimenopausal patients. The active ingredient is usually Nonoxinol. Variations include octoxinol or a polyethoxyethanol derivative.

Special features

The main advantages of chemical contraceptives are their ready availability and ease of application. Strictly, they should always be used in conjunction with the cap, diaphragm or condom, but even used alone they are better than nothing. The high acceptability of chemical products outweighs their relatively high failure rate and in some underdeveloped countries they are likely, therefore, to provide a continuing focus of interest for family-planning programmes. Their effectiveness could undoubtedly be improved by basic research on spermicidal compounds.

SUMMARY

For the patient who requires 100% contraceptive protection, the combined oestrogen–progestogen pills are advised and low-dose (less than 50 μg of oestrogen) preparations should initially be prescribed. Patients refusing to accept or being unsuitable for oestrogen therapy may be offered a single progestogen oral agent.

The oral contraceptive most suited to a particular woman is often found by trial. Some patients are mentally averse to oral contraception and subsequently present with side effects (Table A.7); alternative means of contraception will then be indicated. Regular annual check-ups including cervical smears are mandatory.

Patients declining or being unsuitable for steroid contraceptives may elect an intra-uterine device or barrier method of contraception. Alternatively, should patients have definitively completed their family, a sterilization procedure may be elected.

Table A.7 Possible side effects of oestrogen and progestogen preparations

Oestrogenic effects	Progestogenic effects
Fluid retention and oedema	Breast discomfort
Premenstrual tension and irritability	Depression
Increase in weight associated with oedema	Weight gain associated with increased appetite
Mucorrhoea, cervical erosion	Leucorrhoea, dry vagina
Heavy bleeding	Scanty bleeding
Breakthrough bleeding	Decreased libido
Excessive tiredness	Cramp in legs and abdomen
Vein complaints	Acne, greasy hair
Headache, nausea and vomiting	

Hirsutism

Severe hirsutism in women may be familial or due to an endocrinal abnormality; a full endocrinological assessment should exclude other pathology and careful consideration be given to the risk–benefit ratio before commencing therapy. Cyproterone acetate is recommended for ovarian and adrenal causes of hirsutism.

Ovarian causes:

Polycystic ovarian syndrome
Ovarian stromal hyperplasia
Ovarian hilus cell-hyperplasia

Adrenal cause:

Congenital adrenal hyperplasia

Cyproterone acetate

Cyproterone acetate 2 mg is available as a Pill-type preparation combined with ethinyloestradiol 35 µg, and one tablet is taken daily for 3 weeks out of 4 weeks. It is advocated for patients with idiopathic hirsutism, with severe acne when resistant to antibiotic therapy or as an oral contraceptive in women with androgen-dependent skin conditions.

Presentation

Tablets ethinyloestradiol 35 µg
cyproterone acetate 2 mg

Dose

One tablet daily for 21 days, starting on day 5 of the menstrual cycle.

Contraindications

Acute hepatic disease, malignant disease, severe depression, history of thrombotic disorders.

Side effects

Galactorrhoea and benign breast nodules, sedation and depression, weight gain. Nausea, vomiting, headaches, breast tension, changes in libido and chloasma.

Special features

A prolonged course of therapy may be needed before any improvement is noticed.

Lactation suppression

In the puerperium, for those patients who elect to use artificial foods for their child, lactation may be suppressed using a specific prolactin inhibitor, bromocriptine. Many other drugs suppress lactation and include levodopa, isocarboxazid, phenelzine, tranylcypromine, barbiturates and pyridoxine, but they should not be used clinically for this purpose. However, lactation suppression is only rarely indicated, since measures such as milk expression, breast support and mild analgesics or diuretics will normally suffice. It is reasonable to consider when severe breast engorgement is present and the patient has just delivered a stillborn infant or elected a late mid-trimester abortion.

Alternative drugs are available and include oestrogens (stilboestrol, ethinyloestradiol, quinestrol) (see p. 159) which have met with variable success, but an assocation between deep-vein thrombosis and pulmonary embolism and the suppression of lactation has been noted with stilboestrol, thus reducing the place of oestrogen treatment for the suppression of lactation.

The anti-oestrogens clomiphene citrate and tamoxifen citrate are also effective in suppressing lactation, as is the androgen testosterone enanthate. Norethisterone, 20 mg, 15 mg, 10 mg, 5 mg in a diminishing daily dose, is likewise effective. A serotonin antagonist, metergoline, has also been used. However, it is a dopamine-agonist and stimulates the production of prolactin-inhibiting factor and causes a fall in plasma prolactin concentration.

Dopamine agonists

Bromocriptine mesylate (see p. 54)

The first group of ergot compounds isolated by Barger *et al.* (1906) was called ergotoxine, a mixture of the ergot alkaloids ergocornine, ergocristine and ergocryptine. Bromocriptine (2-bromo-α-ergocryptine) was isolated during research into compounds which inhibited prolactin release without the oxytocic and cardiovascular effects of the parent ergot compound. Bromocriptine is a dopamine agonist; its action on the hypothalamus stimulates production of prolactin-inhibiting factor and it may also act directly, inhibiting the release of prolactin from the pituitary. Hyperprolactinaemia occurs physiologically during pregnancy, when prolactin is involved in developing the mammary gland to its functional state and in promoting and sustaining lactation during the puerperium.

Presentation

Tablets 2.5 mg bromocriptine base.

Dose

Prevention of lactation.	An oral dose of 2.5 mg should be taken on the day of delivery, followed by 2.5 mg twice daily for 14 days.
Suppression of lactation.	An oral dose of 2.5 mg should be taken on the first day, increasing after 2–3 days to twice daily for 14 days.

Contraindications
None known in relationship to the prevention or suppression of lactation.

Indications
It is indicated for the prevention or suppression of lactation (and is also indicated for other hyperprolactinaemic states, for example in hypogonadism and galactorrhoea).

Side effects
These are virtually unknown post-partum. However, the following may occur: nausea (bromocriptine should be taken with food), postural hypotension, dizziness, headache, vomiting and gastrointestinal bleeding. The micturition syncope has also been described. A few isolated cases of hallucinations have been reported. Delayed lactation following the original suppression may occur.

Special features
It does not affect the blood-clotting system. In Europe, another dopamine agonist — lysuride maleate — is also available (see p. 55).

Oestrogens (estrogens)

Quinestrol

This is a derivative of ethinyloestradiol. Oestrogens do not lower prolactin levels; they antagonize the lactogenic activity of prolactin at the breast.

Presentation
Tablets 4 mg.

Dose
A single oral dose of 4–8 mg should be taken within 6 hours of delivery.

Contraindications
These include carcinoma of the breast and reproductive organs or a thrombotic history.

Side effects
If two tablets are used, the patient should be advised that she may experience a heavier than normal period when her menses resume.

Special features
Quinestrol is superior to stilboestrol in preventing rebound lactation in the puerperium (other hormones are in more common use in the United States and include ethinyl estradiol and estradiol valerate, together with testosterone enanthate).

SUMMARY
If a drug is elected to suppress lactation, bromocriptine is the agent of choice. It is best reserved for patients with an intra-uterine or neonatal death in view of its cost.

Further reading

Barger, G., Carr, F.H. and Dale, H.H. (1906). An active alkaloid from ergot. *British Medical Journal*, **2**, 1792.

Carne, S., Chamberlain, G., McEwan, J. (1979). Handbook of Contraceptive practice: International Planner. Parenthood Federation DHSS. London.

Consumers' Association (1992). Mifepristone (Gemeprost) to abort early pregnancy. *Drug and Therapeutics Bulletin*, **31**(2).

Fraser, I.S. (1981). A comprehensive review of injectable contraception with special emphasis on depot medroxyprogesterone acetate. *Medical Journal of Australia*, **1** (1).

Glassier, A. (1993). Drugs in focus: mifepristone. *Prescribers' Journal*, **33**(4), 156–159.

Hawkins, D.F. and Elder, M.G. (1979). *Human Fertility Control*, Butterworths, London.

Inman, W.H.N. and Veasey, M.I. (1968). Investigation of deaths from pulmonary coronary and cerebral thrombosis and embolism in women of childbearing age. *British Medical Journal*, **2**, 190–193.

International Planned Parenthood Federation (1992). Insertable contraception: the USA perspective. *IPPF*, **26** (December).

International Planned Parenthood Federation (1993). International Medical Advisory Panel Statement on Voluntary Surgical Contraception. *IPPF*, **27**(3) (June).

Mascarenha, L. (1994). Long acting methods of contraception. *British Medical Journal*, **308**, 991–992.

Pike, M. (1992). Oral contraceptives and carcinogenesis. Leading article. *Fertility Control and Reviews*, **1**(1), 3–7.

Rall, T.W. and Schleifer, L.S. (1985). *The Pharmacological Basis of Therapeutics. Drugs Affecting Uterine Motility*, 7th edn (eds Goodman and Gilman), Ch. 39, Section 9, p. 926.

Appendix II

Gynaecological Malignancies and Terminal-Care Therapy

Introduction

Some clinical units have attempted to type various gynaecological tumours to different cytotoxic agents, with only limited success, and with the exception of progestogens in the management of endometrial carcinoma and methotrexate in choriocarcinoma, the agents of choice are based on clinical experience. Surgery and radiotherapy remain the mainstay of therapy for malignant disease in gynaecology. Oncological therapy should be guided by specialists, but the general practitioner should be aware of those preparations now being used and the effect their use has on any subsequent prescribing, since interaction between cytotoxics and other drugs can be extremely dangerous. There are many other oncology group protocols in the United States but current drugs and their analogues used in the UK are listed below.

Cytotoxic drugs

Cytotoxic drugs are designed to stop cell division in cancer cells. Normal cells can, however, also be affected and toxic effects noted include nausea and vomiting, alopecia and bone marrow suppression.

1. *Alkylating agents*: **busulphan**, **cyclophosphamide**, **melphalan** and **mustine** — these prevent replication of nucleic acids by cross-linking base pairs. Cyclophosphamide is used in gynaecological cancer; myelosuppression, gastrointestinal disorders and haemorrhagic cystitis are common. *Analogues of alkylating agents*: **treosulfan** is a derivative of busulphan and is used to treat ovarian cancer; it is myelosuppressive and causes skin pigmentation. *Nitrosoureas and their analogues:* these include **carmustine** and **lomustine** and they act as alkylating agents; severe myelosuppression is prolonged and cumulative.

2. *Antimetabolites*: **fluorouracil**, **mercaptopurine**, **methotrexate** — these act by irreversible inhibition of enzyme systems for deoxyribonucleic acid (DNA) or protein synthesis, or by incorporation into nuclear material with subsequent prevention of replication; myelosuppression, mucositis, nephrotoxicity, neurotoxicity and hepatic fibrosis are common. *Analogues of fluorouracil:* several **fluorinated pyrimidines** are under investigation.
3. *Cytotoxic antibiotics*: **actinomycin**, **bleomycin**, **doxorubicin** — these act by intercalation betwen strands of DNA; several analogues of doxorubicin are under investigation to reduce their side effects which include pulmonary fibrosis (bleomycin), alopecia, vomiting and cardiotoxicity (doxorubicin).
4. *Vinca alkaloids and the vinca analogues*: These act by binding to microtubules and preventing metaphase and cell division; vincristine has been used in the management of choriocarcinoma and ovarian malignancy.
5. *New cytotoxic drugs:* (a) **cis-platinum** acts by intercalation of DNA strands — it is used in the treatment of cancer of ovary and cervix; it causes severe gastrointestinal disturbance, myelosuppression, nephrotoxicity and neurotoxicity. (b) **Hexamethylmelamine** is thought to act as both an alkylating agent and antimetabolite; it shows good activity against ovarian cancer and is being tested for cancer of the cervix.cc) **Paclitaxel** was discovered in 1969 in the bark of **Taxus breviflola**, the Pacific Yew Tree; it contains the distinctive taxane ring (see p. 168).

Hormones

These are selective trophic agents that induce specific morphological and functional changes in an organ or tissue. They are mainly used for the treatment of prostatic, breast (tamoxifen) and endometrial cancers (progestogens).

Cytotoxic drugs mainly used in gynaecology are shown in Table A.8. Their side effects are listed in Table A.9.

SPECIFIC GYNAECOLOGICAL CANCERS

Endometrial carcinoma

Progestogens are used in the management of endometrial carcinoma, normally in association with surgery and radiotherapy. Kelly R.M., in 1951, first suggested that sex steroids might control the growth of endometrial carcinoma and, in 1961 showed objective regression in patients treated with progestational agents (Kelly R.M and Baker W.H., 1961).

Table A.8 Drugs used for gynaecological malignancies

Drugs used for gynaecological malignancies
Alkylating agents and analogues
cyclophosphamide, chlorambucil, treosulfan
Antimetabolites
methotrexate
Cytotoxic antibiotics
bleomycin, doxorubicin
New cytotoxic drugs
cis-platinum
paclitaxel
Hormones
progestogens

Table A.9 Side effects of cytotoxic drugs

Cytotoxic drugs are selective with a low therapeutic index; they tend to be used in toxic dosages, and common side effects expected include:

Local effects: thrombophlebitis, cellulitis
Nausea and vomiting
Marrow suppression
Hair loss — cyclophosphamide
Mouth ulceration — methotrexate
Neurotoxicity — cis-platinum
Cardiotoxicity — doxorubicin
Lung toxicity — bleomycin
Skin disorders — bleomycin

Gestronol hexanoate (17-hexanoyloxy-19-norpregn-4-ene-3, 20-dione)
This is a depot progestogen and is 25 times more potent than its parent substance, progesterone. Its action is concentrated on the endometrium, acting directly without pituitary suppression.

Presentation
Injection 200 mg/2ml.

Dose
(a) *To inhibit metastatic spread before and after surgery:* 200–400 mg should be given intramuscularly every 5–7 days; treatment should commence immediately

following the diagnosis and be continued for a minimum of 12 weeks. (b) *To treat metastases:* 200–400 mg should be given intramuscularly every 5–7 days and continued for as long as required.

Contraindications
A history of herpes in pregnancy is a contraindication.

Side effects
Local reactions may occur at the injection site, exacerbation may occur in bronchial asthma, epilepsy and migraine, and there may be a moderate rise in serum liver enzymes.

Special features
In patients with chronic liver damage, it is advisable to check liver function during long-term treatment.

Medroxyprogesterone acetate, BP, USP
This is an oral progestogen.

Presentation
Tablets   100 mg, 200 mg, 400 mg.

Dose
An oral dose of 200–400 mg should be taken daily for up to 3 months; variable dose regimes apply 400 mg–1.5 g daily may also be used.

Contraindications
Liver disease; thromboembolic disease.

Indications
It is used to treat metastases in endometrial carcinoma. It may be given prophylactically to inhibit metastatic spread before or after surgery.

Side effects
It has a corticosteroid-like effect, reducing adrenal response; mastodynia, galactorrhoea, weight gain and mild oedema may occur.

Special features
Medroxyprogesterone acetate is also used in the management of secondary dysmenorrhoea, (see p. 65) and progestogen-only contraceptive (see p. 152). It should be used cautiously where there is a history of depression, diabetes, epilepsy, migraine, asthma or cardiac or renal dysfunction.

Hydatidiform mole/choriocarcinoma

The treatment of these conditions is monitored by radioimmunoassay of human chorionic gonadotrophin levels, and regional specialist centres have been established. Although methotrexate is the agent of choice, other drugs have been used for these conditions including actinomycin D, cyclophosphamide, vincristine and cytosine arabinoside.

Methotrexate, BP, Eur.P, USP

This antimetabolite acts by competitive inhibition with the enzyme dihydrofolate reductase. It inhibits reduction of folic acid and interferes with tissue cell reproduction.

Presentation

Tablets 2.5 mg.

Dose

One suggested regimen is methotrexate 0.25–1 mg/kg body weight (up to maximum of 60 mg) by intramuscular injection every 48 hours for four doses. Leucovorin 6 mg is given by intramuscular injection every 48 hours for four doses, 30 hours after each injection of methotrexate. A 7-day rest interval is allowed between the last day of one course of methotrexate and the first day of the next course, but may be extended depending on haematological toxity. The leucovorin should be increased to 9 mg intramuscularly if significant stomatitis occurs at the lower dose level. This regimen does, however, minimize gastrointestinal, dermatological and haematological side effects. Patients who are considered to be 'medium or high risk' need to be treated from the start of chemotherapy with combination regimens. Inappropriate treatment jeopardizes the patient's chance of care.

Contraindications

These include pregnancy, hepatic and renal impairment and blood dyscrasias, unless the benefits of therapy outweight the associated risks.

Side effects

Diarrhoea or ulcerative stomatitis, haemorrhagic enteritis and death from intestinal perforation, and bone-marrow depression with pancytopenia, may all occur. It is hepatotoxic.

Special features

An enhanced effect occurs with aminobenzoic acid, salicylates, sulphonamides and thiazide diuretics. Methotrexate for intrathecal use is not available in the United States. Strict monitoring is essential including: haematology, urine analysis, renal function tests and liver-function tests. Methotrexate interacts with protein-bound drugs, alcohol, live vaccines, folic acid, etretinate, anticonvulsants, non-steroidal anti-inflammatory drugs, penicillin, co-trimoxazole, trimethoprim, cyclosporin, antimalarials and uricosurics.

Carcinoma of the ovary

Whilst progestogens have been used for ovarian malignancy, more specific cytotoxics are available for this condition, including the alkylating agents chlorambucil, cyclophosphamide and treosulfan which is said to be especially effective in controlling ascites. The antibiotic doxorubicin has also been used in the management of ovarian cancer and newer agents include cis-platinum and paclitaxel.

Alkylating agents

Chlorambucil, BP, USP

Although some authors consider this as the drug of choice for carcinoma of the ovary, others state that there is very little to choose between the various alkylating agents.

Presentation

Tablets 2 mg, 5 mg

Dose

An oral dose of 200 µg/kg body weight should be taken daily for 4–6 weeks.

Contraindications

As for other antimitotic agents (see below).

Side effects

As for other antimitotic agents (see below).

Special features

Chlorambucil does not cause alopecia.

Cyclophosphamide, BP, USP

This drug, as with all alkylating agents, interferes with normal mitoses and cell division in all rapidly proliferating tissue.

Presentation

Injection	(anhydrous cyclophosphamide)	100 mg, 200 mg, 500 mg, 1 g
Tablets	50 mg	

Dose

Many variations are available, but one suggested regimen is: day 1, 50 mg should be given by intravenous injection; days 2–9, 100 mg; day 10, 150 mg; then treatment is continued with 50 mg twice daily orally.

Contraindications

These include chronic inflammatory suppuration, pancytopenia.

Indications

It is advised in the management of carcinoma of the ovary (and other malignancies which are sensitive to cyclophosphamide).

Side effects

These include alopecia and bone marrow depression (the white-cell count, platelet and haemoglobin levels should be monitored), cystitis and nausea and vomiting. Haematuria and urothelial toxicity.

Special features

This drug has been given in a multi-drug regime, including vincristine, procarbazine hydrochloride, prednisolone and other cytotoxic agents. Combination therapy increases the side effects. It has also been used as adjuvant therapy during surgery. It interacts with radiotherapy, doxorubicin and sulphonylureas.

New cytotoxic drugs

Platinum diamminodichloride (cis-platinum)

This is indicated as palliative therapy, used in addition to other modalities, or in established combination therapy for metastatic ovarian tumours.

Presentation

Vials 10 mg, 50 mg, 100 mg,

Dose

A single intravenous dose of 50–120 mg/m^2 body surface every 3–4 weeks or a daily intravenous dose of 15–20 mg/m^2 body surface for 5 days every 3–4 weeks. With combination therapy, lower doses ranging from 20 mg/m^2 body surface upwards, administered intravenously, every 3–4 weeks are used.

Contraindications

Hypersensitivity to platinum-containing compounds. Pregnancy and breast-feeding mothers. Hyperuricaemia and hypomagnaseaemia.

Side effects

Platinum diamminodichloride induces nephrotoxicity, myelosuppression, neurotoxicity and ototoxicity. Anaphylactic-type reactions have been reported.

Special features

Platinum diamminodichloride should be administered by individuals experienced in the use of antineoplastic therapy. A pretreatment hydration with 1–2 litres of fluid infused for 8–12 hours prior to a platinum diamminodichloride dose is recommended, in order to initiate diuresis and adequate hydration, and urinary output maintained for 24 hours following administration. Peripheral blood counts should be monitored weekly, audiometric testing and renal function studies performed prior to therapy and the absence of symptoms of peripheral neuropathy established prior to therapy.

Paclitaxel

Paclitaxel acts by promoting the assembly of microtubules from tubulin dimers and stabilizing microtubules by preventing depolymerization. This inhibits the normal functioning of microtubules during mitosis (where microtubules function as part of the mitotic spindle apparatus), as well as during interphase. In addition, paclitaxel causes the formation of abnormal arrays or 'bundles' of microtubules throughout the cell cycle, and multiple asters of microtubules during mitosis.

Indications

It can be of value for platinum-resistant cancers but should be administered in experienced oncology centres.

Dose

175 mg/m^2 over 3 hours every 3 weeks.

Side effects

Neutropenia; thrombocytopenia anaemia.

Carcinoma of the cervix

Doxorubicin hydrochloride, USP

This is an anthracycline antibiotic which displays activity against a wide range of human neoplasms including a variety of solid tumour; unfortunately the clinical value is limited by an unusual cardiomyopathy.

Presentation

Vials 10 mg, 50 mg

Dose

This is calculated on the basis of body surface area: 60–75 mg/m^2 may be given every 3 weeks when used alone; in combination therapy, the dose is reduced to 30–40 mg/m^2 every 3 weeks; based on body weight, the dose 1.2—2.4 mg/kg should be given as a single dose every 3 weeks. A weekly dose of 20 mg/m^2 is as effective as a 3 weekly regime and reduces cardiotoxicity.

Contraindications

Bone-marrow depression or buccal ulceration or premonitory buccal burning; sedation; impaired cardiac function; pregnancy and breast-feeding mothers.

Side effects

Bone-marrow depression; alopecia, nausea, vomiting and diarrhoea; red coloration of urine; irreversible congestive cardiac failure with cumulative doses of more than 550 mg/m^2 body surface.

Special features
The normal dosage should be reduced in the presence of liver impairment. The drug should be used under the direction of those experienced in cytotoxic therapy.

SUMMARY
Cytotoxic therapy is of proven value with endometrial carcinoma, choriocarcinoma and carcinoma of the ovary. It is, as yet, of limited value for carcinoma of the cervix. Carcinoma of the vagina and vulva should be treated surgically but radiotherapy can be considered. All agents have serious side effects, and strict monitoring of therapy is mandatory.

Terminal-care therapy (see Chapter 8)

Drugs are a useful adjuvant to the expertise of good medical and nursing care for terminal-care management. The opiates pethidine, morphine and diamorphine should be liberally prescribed to relieve pain and for sedation. Other useful drugs include the non-steroidal anti-inflammatory analgesics, corticosteroids, psychotropics, anticonvulsants and the central-acting analgesics.

Morphine is available as slow-release tablets in strengths of 10 mg, 30 mg, 60 mg and 100 mg and diamorphine is available as dispersible diamorphine tablets 10 mg. Either drug may be used in single mixtures with chloroform water; e.g. morphine hydrochloride 5 mg, chloroform water to 5 ml.

Intractable pelvic pain may be relieved by single-shot intra-arterial administration of cytotoxic drugs, e.g. nitrogen mustard, or epidural or caudal blocks using phenol. Chordotomy may be required.

In addition to the relief of pain, supportive measures including anti-emetic therapy (Table A.10) will be indicated and whereas routine metoclopramide hydrochloride or the phenothiazines including promethazine theoclate, chlorpromazine hydrochloride or thiethylperazine maleate may be selected, other anti-emetics are available for vomiting secondary to cytotoxic therapy, including betahistine hydrochloride, cinnarizine, cyclizine, domperidone, nabilone and 5-HT$_3$-antagonists which block the effects of dopamine released from the chemoreceptor trigger zone and also increase lower oesophageal sphincter pressure and improve delayed gastric emptying. They are free from central side effects.

Table A.10 Anti-emetics

Antihistamines
- cyclizine hydrochloride
- cinnarizine
- dimenhydrinate
- promethazine theoclate
- prochlorperazine maleate
- trifluoperazine hydrochloride
- methotrimeprazine

Anticholinergic drugs — hyoscine

Cannabinoids — nabilone

Dopamine antagonists
- phenothiazines
- metoclopramide
- domperidone

5-HT_3 antagonists
- granisetron
- ondansetron
- tropisetron

Domperidone

This is a peripherally acting dopamine antagonist.

Presentation

Tablets	10 mg	
Suspension	1 mg/ml	on a named patient basis only
Injection	5 mg/ml	on a named patient basis only
Suppositories	30 mg	on a named patient basis only

Dose

An oral dose of one-to-two tablets or 10 mg by intramuscular or intravenous use at 4–8 hourly intervals: or one-to-two suppositories rectally, 4–8 hourly.

Contraindications

Pregnancy.

Special features

Cardiac dysrhythmias may occur after an intravenous bolus and patients should receive an infusion rather than an intravenous bolus, diluted 1:10 in saline, given over 15–30 minutes. The parenteral form is available from the manufacturer on a named patient basis.

Ondansetron hydrochloride

This is a 5-HT_3 antagonist. It has potent anti-emetic actions and is also used for post-operative nausea and vomiting.

Presentation

Tablets	4.0 mg, 8.0 mg
Injection	2 mg/ml, 2 ml, 4 ml

Dose

8.0 mg by slow intravenous injection immediately before treatment or orally 1 hour before treatment and 8.0 mg orally every 12 hours for 5 days. The efficacy can be enhanced by dexamethasone 20 mg i.v. and the dose can be tailored by personal experience of the clinician.

Special features

Constipation, headache, flushing can all occur.

Nabilone

This is a cannabinoid and it is thought to have a central effect involving opiate receptors.

Presentation

1 mg tablets.

Dose

Usually 1 mg twice daily rising to 2 mg twice daily up to a maximum daily dose of 6 mg (2 mg tds). The first dose is administered the night before starting chemotherapy. The second dose is administered 1–3 hours prior to chemotherapy. Continue for 48 hours after the last dose of chemotherapy if necessary.

Contraindications

Patients with a known allergy to cannabinoid agents. When nausea and vomiting arises from any cause other than cancer chemotherapy. It is excreted primarily by biliary route and is not recommended in patients with severe liver disease. May impair mental and physical abilities (caution operating machinery). CNS effects persist for a variable time post dose (up to 72 hours). Can cause mood changes and adverse behavioural effects. Can elevate supine and standing heart rate, cause postural hypotension – caution in elderly and patients with hypertension/heart disease. Use with caution in patients taking other psychoactive drugs or those with history of psychiatric disorders. Has additive depressant effect when given with barbiturates, benzodiazepines, alcohol and narcotics.

Side effects

Nearly all patients experience at least one of the folowing: psychomimetic reactions, drowsiness, vertigo, euphoria, dry mouth, ataxia, visual disturbances, dysphoria, hypotension, headache, nausea, confusion, disorientation, hallucination, psychosis, depression, decreased co-ordination, tremors, tachycardia, decreased appetite and abdominal pain.

Special features

Not to be administered to those under 18 years old. Nabilone is abusable, capable of producing a euphoria at therapeutic doses. Prescribing should be limited to the few days necessary for chemotherapy cycle. Signs and symptoms of overdosage are an extension of psychomimetric side effects and can occur at prescribed doses – withold further doses until mental state returned to base line mental status (up to 72 hours). Monitor 'vital signs' since hypo- and hypertension can occur as can tachycardia and general supportive care.

Further reading

Kelly, R.M. and Baker, W.H. (1961). Progestational agents in the treatment of carcinoma of endometrium. *New England Journal of Medicine*, **264**, 216–222.

Rowinski, E.K., Onetto, N., Canetta, R.M. *et al.* (1992). Taxol: the first of the taxanes, an important new class of anti-tumour agents. *Seminars in Oncology*, **19**, 646–662.

Smith, G. and Rowbotham, D.J. (1992). Postoperative nausea and vomiting. *British Journal of Anaesthesia*, **69**(7) (Suppl. 1).

Vickers, M.D. (1992). Ondansetron — Postoperative nausea and vomiting. *European Journal of Anaesthesiology*, Supplement 6.

Wani, M.C., Taylor, H.L., Wall, M.E. *et al.* (1971). Plant antitumour agents, The isolation and structure of taxol — a novel antileukaemic and antitumour agent from *Taxus brevifolia*. *Journal of the American Chemical Society*, **93**, 2325–2327.

Index

Note: Page numbers in *italics* refer to tables